AF609599

THE ELECTRONIC HEALTH RECORDS SPECIALIST

Focusing on the Role for Organizational Success

Maria Revell

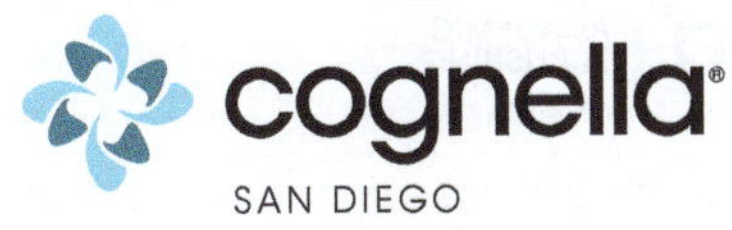

Bassim Hamadeh, CEO and Publisher
Amanda Martin, Executive Publisher
Amy Smith, Associate Editorial Manager
Abbey Hastings, Senior Production Editor
Emely Villavicencio, Senior Graphic Designer
Kylie Bartolome, Licensing Specialist
Natalie Piccotti, Director of Marketing
Kassie Graves, Senior Vice President, Editorial
Alia Bales, Director, Project Editorial and Production

Copyright © 2025 by Cognella, Inc. All rights reserved. No part of this publication may be reprinted, reproduced, transmitted, or utilized in any form or by any electronic, mechanical, or other means, now known or hereafter invented, including photocopying, microfilming, and recording, or in any information retrieval system without the written permission of Cognella, Inc. For inquiries regarding permissions, translations, foreign rights, audio rights, and any other forms of reproduction, please contact the Cognella Licensing Department at rights@cognella.com.

Trademark Notice: Product or corporate names may be trademarks or registered trademarks and are used only for identification and explanation without intent to infringe.

Cover image: Copyright © 2020 iStockphoto LP/metamorworks.

Printed in the United States of America.

This book is designed to provide educational information and motivation to our readers. It is sold with the understanding that the publisher is not engaged to render any type of psychological, legal, diet, health, exercise or any other kind of professional advice. The content of each chapter or reading is the sole expression and opinion of its author, and not necessarily that of the publisher. No warranties or guarantees are expressed or implied by the publisher's choice to include any of the content in this volume. Neither the publisher nor the individual author(s) shall be liable for any physical, psychological, emotional, financial, or commercial damages, including, but not limited to, special, incidental, consequential or other damages. Our views and rights are the same: You are responsible for your own choices, actions, and results and for seeking relevant topical advice from trained professionals.

The author generated Chapter Summaries 1-10 in part with GPT-3.5, OpenAI's large-scale language-generation model. Upon generating draft language, the author reviewed, further researched, edited, and revised most language to their own liking and takes ultimate responsibility for this content in the publication. Any direct content used is referenced herein.

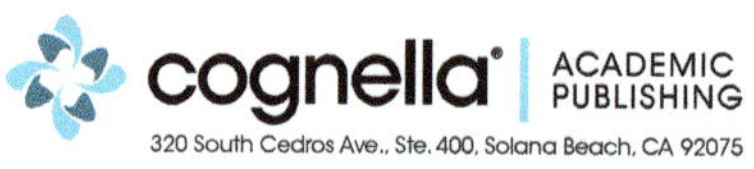

Brief Contents

Detailed Contents

CHAPTER 4

Health Care Settings and Personnel 27

CHAPTER 5

Laws and Regulations Governing EHRs 34

CHAPTER 11

EHRS Certification Test Plan Specific Information 110

Preface

This book, *The Electronic Health Records Specialist: Focusing on the Role for Organizational Success*, came from my desire to promote a successful educational outcome for others. Education has been part of my life's work for over 35 years. The book holistically addresses the role of the electronic health records specialist (EHRS) from who they are to expectations for their job and basic requirements, such as knowledge of abbreviations and medical terms. It promotes self-growth and focuses on the role of the EHRS as a member of the organizational team. It emphasizes how integration into this role is required for organizational success. This book will help the student navigate the landscape of being in the role of an EHRS and move their organization to success.

There is growing importance for the role of an EHRS as there is an increasing dependence on technology in health care. This is driven by new regulations that affect reimbursement for providers and organizations such as promoting interoperability programs. It has also been driven by the many nonauthorized intrusive episodes of data capture for ransom from outside organizational entities. The EHRS has become an integral part of a successful health care organization as they enhance patient care delivery, streamline processes for data capture and system integration, and facilitate data-driven decisions for hospitals and clinics. This is not a role that can just be taken by an individual without proper education and training, as implementation of the EHR is complex and multifaceted. Educational success is facilitated in the book by inclusion of pedagogical aids such as chapter objectives, key terms, headings for information transition, appropriate tables and figures, and chapter summaries. This book is designed to facilitate a student's positive outcome.

I wish all who use this book much success in their educational endeavors!

Maria A. Revell, PhD, MSN, RN, COI
2024

Reviewers

Marcia A. Pugh, DNP, MSN, MBA, HCM, RN

Charles W. Revell, MCP, MCAD, MCSD, MCT

JLynn Jennifer Brown, MSL, RHIA, CPCO, CDEI, CPB, CMRS, CMCS, AHI (AMT), RMA (AMT), HITCM-PP

Neosho County Community College

Kristy Courville, MHA, RHIA

University of Louisiana at Lafayette

Larena Grieshaber

Northeast State Community College

1

THE ELECTRONIC HEALTH RECORDS SPECIALIST

CHAPTER OBJECTIVES

Upon completion of this chapter, the reader will be able to do the following:

1. Define the *Electronic Health Records Specialist* (EHRS).
2. Identify the role of the EHRS in an organization.
3. Support the use of an analytical problem-solving approach for the EHRS.
4. Demonstrate steps the EHRS can use for problem solving.
5. Document skills needed by the EHRS.

KEY CHAPTER TERMS

- Electronic health record (EHR)
- Electronic Health Records Specialist (EHRS)
- Implementation and Optimization Specialist role
- Training and Education Coordinator role
- System Administrator role
- Quality Assurance Analyst role
- Compliance Officer role
- Interoperability Specialist role
- Technical skills (computer skill proficiency)
- Analytical skills (problem-solving capability)
- Interpersonal skills (effective communication)

The EHR and the Specialist

The Electronic Health Record (EHR) is a lifelong technological copy of a patient or client's medical history that is maintained by the health care provider over the care delivery timeframe. It can include numerous components such as demographic data, notes regarding care progress, medical diagnoses for problems identified, biological data (laboratory results and assessment information), and so forth. Although many organizations completely use electronic systems, some smaller clinics and organizations may combine parts of the electronic system with the use of paper portions (hybrid system) of the patient health record. Verification of the EHR is an important part of patient data retrieval as this allows for identification of new problems or the need for continuation of care for existing problems.

Electronic Health Records Specialist (EHRS) duties will depend on the size and specialty of the organization. If the organization has an information technology (IT) department, it will be critical for the EHRS to work in collaboration with this department to perform their duties. In addition to just keeping records, responsibilities may also include compiling care and census data, working with researchers for data retrieval from patient records, working with department managers to develop or revise policies related to patient records, and assisting with daily office operations.

Role of the Electronic Health Records Specialist

The EHRS is a critical member of the healthcare team and must be able to effectively work with other health care professionals in the provision of high-quality care to all patients. They play a crucial role in the health care industry by managing and maintaining records and systems. Responsibilities of someone in this role are varied and can include data management, education, interoperability, and compliance based on organization size and objectives (see Figure 1.1).

- The *Implementation and Optimization Specialist* role is responsible for overseeing EHR deployment within various organizations. This includes conducting needs assessments to understand organizational requirements for effective functioning and workflow, collaborating with stakeholders to select appropriate EHR solutions, configuring systems,

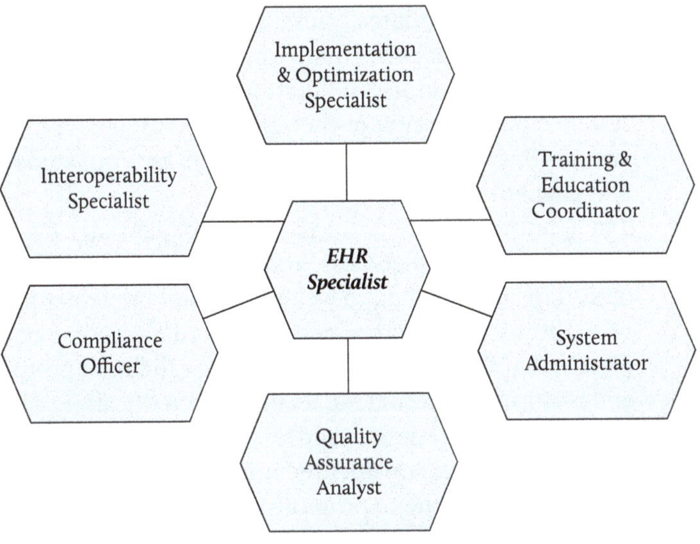

FIGURE 1.1 Role of the EHRS.

developing implementation and ongoing optimization plans, and providing ongoing support. This ensures successful adoption, implementation, and ongoing effective system upgrades for proper functioning and organizational support.

- The ***Training and Education Coordinator* role** involves developing and delivering specialist training needs to staff in system management and use. This includes developing training materials that address specific user groups such as manuals, tutorials, and interactive modules; delivery of initial or refresher educational offerings either in person or virtually; and collaborating with subject matter experts to develop materials related to specific care areas or detailed unique workflows. These educational activities ensure that staff know how to navigate the system interface to support safe and effective patient care delivery.
- The ***System Administrator* role** manages and maintains EHR day-to-day requirements. This includes managing user access and permissions to ensure compliance with organizational and security policies and regulations; monitoring system performance and troubleshooting and resolving issues; performing routine maintenance tasks

such as system updates, backups, and system patches for continued system performance and reliability; and collaborating with vendors and technology support to ensure system enhancements are effectively implemented. This role ensures that the organizational EHR system runs smoothly and efficiently.

- The ***Quality Assurance Analyst* role** focuses on ensuring the accuracy, completeness, and reliability of EHR system data. This role includes development and implementation of quality assurance processes to ensure data accuracy, completeness and consistency; establishing validation protocols and performing checks for data integrity verification; collaborating with end users to address identified quality issues, providing feedback on documentation reviews and offering any needed training to promote continued data entry best practices; generating reports on data quality metrics; and participating in audits and assessments. This role ensures demonstration of organizational compliance with relevant standards and regulations.
- The ***Compliance Officer* role** confirms that organizational EHR systems adhere to relevant regulations, standards, and industry best practices. This role accomplishes its intent through the development and maintenance of current policies, procedures, and documentation to support regulatory compliance and adherence to industry best practices; the provision of training and educational offerings on compliance requirements, data privacy, and recommended corrective actions; collaboration with legal counsel and regulatory agencies to address compliance issues, respond to inquiries, address audit concerns, and mitigate risks; and monitor regulatory changes and industry standards that affect current EHR systems and organizational processes. This role ensures compliance with laws such as the Health Insurance Portability and Accountability Act (HIPAA) and reduces compliance risks.
- The ***Interoperability Specialist* role** facilities the exchange of health information between EHR systems and other health care IT systems. This role ensures seamless integration and data sharing across differing platforms. The role monitors interface performance, troubleshoots connectivity issues, and implements enhancements; implements and maintains

interfaces between the EHR and other organizational IT systems; ensures compliance with interoperability standards; and provides training and support to end users regarding interoperability workflows, protocols for data sharing, and information exchange best practices. This promotes coordination of care and interoperability among interprofessional and intra-professional health care team members.

Smaller organizations, clinics, and offices may combine the roles of employees and staff such as Medical Administrative Assistant/Electronic Medical Records Specialist. Administrative assistants may be identified by other titles such as office manager/assistant, administrative specialist/support, office supervisor, and so on.

Administrative Assistant Roles may be combined in part or fully with EHRS responsibilities:

- checking patients in at the front desk
- answering the phone or responding to electronic communications
- scheduling appointments
- interviewing patients to obtain demographic and case histories information prior to a health care appointment
- compiling medical records and charts
- processing insurance payments
- operating various computer software programs and other office equipment
- validating receipt and transfer of laboratory results to the appropriate health care provider
- maintaining supplies and professional appearance of the office

EHRS roles may include the following:

- analyzing patient records for completeness and compliance
- ensuring that records are stored securely and in compliance with regulations
- capturing key administrative and clinical data elements from records for reports
- performing basic coding to submit reimbursement claims
- processing Release of Information (ROI) requests for medical records

- reviewing patient records to ensure completion and accuracy
- collecting patient demographic and insurance information
- discussing patient information with health care providers and insurance professionals

Management of records requires critical skills. Knowledge of health care regulations is required, which includes HIPAA, an underlying premise for all interactions. There are several federal requirements that must be adhered to in order to maintain the office in compliance. These specific regulations are addressed later in the book.

EHRS Skills

The role of the EHRS includes a strong foundation in various skills, which include **technical skills (computer skill proficiency)**, **analytical skills (problem-solving capability)**, and **interpersonal skills (effective communication)** (see Figure 1.2).

Computer skills proficiency with software programs complements EHRS duties. Knowledge and the ability to understand relevant programs are needed for processing text and numerical data. The EHR specialist may be required to customize systems and perform system upgrades and maintenance. Keeping the system up-to-date provides for proper hardware and software functioning.

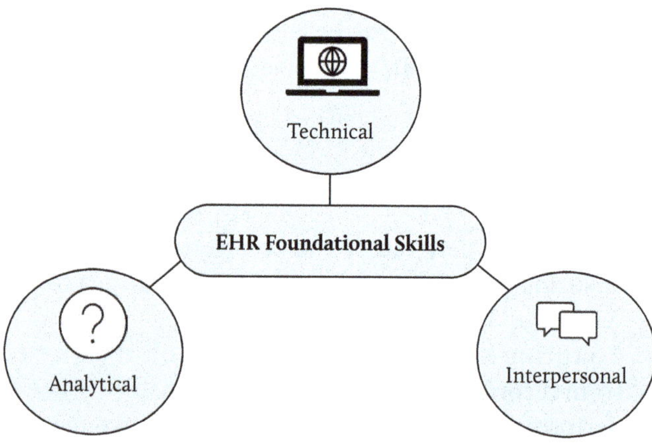

FIGURE 1.2 EHRS skills.

Since the EHRS works with forms and workflows, they may also be responsible for customizing these and configuring system specifics related to both templates and forms. These combined with analytical skills allow the EHRS to analyze retrieved data and identify trends or issues that require attention and intervention to meet goals and outcomes.

Communication is important to effectively address and deal with patients, coworkers, and others in a professional manner. This quality is needed in all forms of communication, face-to-face, verbally, and in writing over various formats to include audio (phones) and electronic devices (via video, email, and chat).

Problem Solving

Problem solving is important in many jobs, and the EHRS is no different. Having the ability to go through a problem-solving process to identify and address issues can lead to a reduction in downtime and loss of revenue. The use of an analytical problem-solving approach can facilitate efficient problem identification and resolution for promoting a continuous workflow. There are several problem-solving processes, and this is just one that can be effectively used for problem resolution.

There are many ways to achieve an outcome after going through a problem-solving process, which can include a four-step to a seven-step process. Table 1.1 shows a five-step process that combines some of the seven steps but may be easy to remember in looking at a viable way to problem solve.

TABLE 1.1 Steps in a Problem-Solving Process (Five Steps)

Steps	Processes to Achieve the Step
1. Define the problem.	1. Exactly what is the problem? Look at the facts, not the opinions of self or others. 2. Write down the problem. Read and reread the problem statement to clearly understand what has been violated or what expectation was not met.

(*Continued*)

TABLE 1.1 *(Continued)*

Steps	Processes to Achieve the Step
2. Generate solutions for the problem.	1. Identify if you can solve the problem yourself or if you need to include others in looking for a solution. 2. Look at solutions that may have already been used as a solution to this problem. 3. Consider alternatives that meet organizational goals and objectives that will solve the problem. 4. Make a list of possible solutions.
3. Evaluate and select a solution.	1. Carefully examine each solution critically, analyzing them without bias or opinion. 2. Select one solution that meets organizational goals and objectives (usually the simplest solution is easiest to implement and requires fewer resources and less time). 3. Select one solution that can be implemented (you / the organization have the ability, time, resources, and cost to implement). 4. Break the solution down into steps for implementation.
4. Implement solution.	1. Plan the implementation process. Approach may be all at once or incremental (gradually over a period of time). 2. Monitor and collect information/data that gives you a clear picture of success or failure.
5. Evaluate the solution and revise as needed.	1. Analyze information/data collected. 2. Identify if the problem was solved using the decided solution. 3. Revise proposed solution if it did not solve the identified problem. It may be necessary to start the process over if the problem has changed or there have been changes to organizational goals or objectives that conflict with the original proposed solution.

Chapter Summary

The EHRS is an important member of the collaborative health care professional team responsible for managing and optimizing organizational electronic health record systems. Their role involves ensuring the accurate documentation, secure storage, and efficient utilization of patient health information for organizational support. It is important for the EHRS to use a problem-solving approach to identify, analyze, and resolve issues related to the EHR system to maintain workflow and accurate data quality. The EHRS must have a strong foundation in combined technical, analytical, and interpersonal skills to effectively manage the system. These are required to ensure the delivery of high-quality patient care by a collaborative health care team.

CREDIT

Fig. 1.2a: Icons are Copyright © by Microsoft.

2

THE EHR HISTORY AND TIMELINE

CHAPTER OBJECTIVES

Upon completion of this chapter, the reader will be able to do the following:

1. Discuss the EHR history.
2. Identify the EHR evolution timeline.
3. Describe the timeline for EHR adoption components of HIPAA and Health Information Technology for Economic and Clinical Health (HI-TECH) Act.
4. Differentiate between the EHR and an Electronic Medical Record (EMR).
5. Evaluate the use of the personal health record in patient health care management.

KEY CHAPTER TERMS

- EHR evolution
- Institute of Medicine
- Electronic Health Record
- Electronic Medical Record
- Personal Health Record

EHR History

The EHR evolved over many years and has involved numerous organizations and industries to get to its current state. The EHR history helps us understand the changes that have occurred over these many years. Prior years formed the foundation for current systems as these current systems will form the foundation for future ones. These evolutionary transitions promoted progression of the EHR, and understanding this past perspective gives us insight and an appreciation for current emerging changes in the EHR.

The **electronic health record (EHR)** was initiated in the 1960s. Medical centers and hospitals began using computerized information systems to manage patient data during this time period. It was not until 30 years later, in the 1990s, that this terminology was used.

The **Institute of Medicine (IOM)** published "The Computer-Based Patient Record: An Essential Technology for Health Care" in 1991. This report called for the widespread implementation of the EHR to improve the quality of health care and reduce overall health care costs.

The IOM identified benefits of improved patient safety, reduced medical errors, and increased efficacy of health care delivery. One of the biggest potentials identified was the ability of the EHR to promote information exchange between interdisciplinary health care providers. With one record containing all patient information, this could facilitate clinical decision-making based on complete and accurate patient data.

A vision of the report identified a comprehensive, integrated, and accessible patient record accessible across the health care system. This has partially been achieved to date as no unified nationwide system exists. Although there are systems that are accessible, these are separate and generally contained within one organization requiring patients to sign waivers for access to records in other computerized data software systems. The IOM report identified technical and organizational challenges that needed to be addressed in order for the vision of unification of records to be realized. These challenges included the need for interoperability between different systems, data format standardization, and robust data security and privacy for records in the program.

The report brought to the forefront the need for computer-based patient records. This data automation would not only modernize health care delivery but promote widespread adoption to improve quality of care and reduce consumer costs.

In 2004, a goal to have EHRs for all Americans by 2014 was set by President George W. Bush. The American Recovery and Reinvestment Act (ARRA) in 2009 included provisions for implementation as part of a larger effort to modernize health care delivery.

The EHR is a computerized lifelong health care record for patients that can track care across decades, providers, and organizations. Today you will see the EHR used by health care providers worldwide. Research has validated that they improve patient safety, reduce medical errors, including medication errors, and increase health care delivery efficiency by an interdisciplinary team of providers. The EHR is especially useful in promoting disease management for individuals with chronic illnesses. Challenges persist despite the many changes that have been made in computerized data software programs to facilitate ease of data entry and access. These include (a) interoperability between the different EHR systems and (b) privacy and security concerns for data in systems that have the potential to be compromised.

EHR Evolution Timeline

The **EHR evolution** began in the 1960s and continues to evolve and transform the health care industry. Figure 2.1 is a timeline for this evolution.

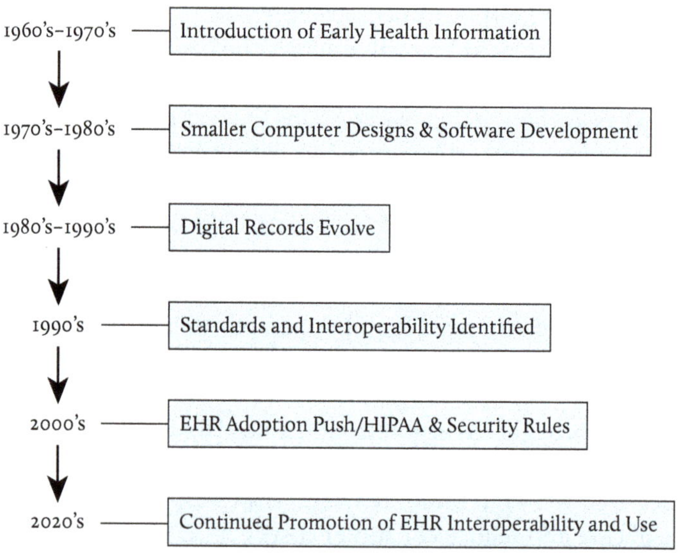

FIGURE 2.1 EHR evolution.

1960s to 1970s: Early health information systems come on the scene.

- Computers developed that could maintain records in an electronic format, but they were large and required space and specialized personnel expertise to run and manage. Mainframe purchase and management were required, which expensed these outside the affordable range of many health care organizations.

1970s to 1980s: Smaller computer designs and software development

- Computer technology advances with software designed for specific health care organizational use. Computer use expanded to include department-specific functions such as pharmacy, the clinical laboratory, billing, and patient registration. These activities were still siloed within departments, which meant they could not be easily accessed.

1980s to 1990s: Digital records evolve

- Many health care organizations began in earnest to transition from paper to electronic records as EHR systems developed and grew in capability. This was accentuated by a 1983 amendment of the Social Security Act to include a Diagnosis Related Group (DRG) patient classification system that identified a hospital prospective payment system for all Medicare patients. This required many health care organizations to link financial and clinical systems to validate payment reimbursement. This was accomplished to a limited degree.

1990s: Identification of standards and interoperability

- With the evolution of more compact, powerful, and affordable hardware and software, use increased and standards were developed. HIPAA was signed into law.

2000s: EHR Adoption Push and HIPAA Privacy and Security Rules

- The Health Information Technology for Economic and Clinical Health (HITECH) Act incentivized health care providers to implement EHRs with the Meaningful Use incentive program. This was later replaced with the Promoting Interoperability Program.

- The final privacy rule was published, where Protected Health Information (PHI) was defined and stipulations for use and disclosure were identified.
- The Enforcement Rule of March 2006 explained how the Department of Health and Human Services would investigate and issue monetary penalties for failure to comply with the Privacy Rule.
- The final Omnibus Rule of 2013 specified encryption standards required to make electronic PHI unreadable, unusable, and undecipherable in the event of an organization's health information system breech.

2020s: Continued promotion of EHR interoperability and use

- Continued efforts to improve interoperability. Focus on data exchange between various health care organization systems and different providers. Introduction of technological advances into health care systems to enhance decision-making such as machine learning and the use of artificial intelligence. Technological advancements allow for incorporation of data and algorithms for decision-making for tasks to promote better patient outcomes.
- Response to the coronavirus disease 2019 (COVID-19) pandemic increased EHR use and highlighted the need for these systems to be able to retrieve data from various outside entities. The COVID-19 pandemic stressed the need for EHR systems to be able to respond to public health emergencies and resulted in the development of improved system interoperability.

Difference Between the Electronic Health Record and Electronic Medical Record

EHR and Electronic Medical Record (EMR) are often used interchangeably, but they are very different in scope and purpose (see Table 2.1). The EHR is broad in scope because it integrates or merges information from multiple health care providers and organizations with interoperability. This allows synchronization of information and data from different systems to enhance care coordination and therefore improve outcomes on a larger scale. The EHR includes clinical, laboratory, pharmacies, insurer, and so forth information for the patient. This gives a comprehensive view of the patient's entire health care history over time from various providers in diverse settings.

The EMR is more confined in its scope in that it only provides information from one health care provider or a single health care organization. This digital patient record is used primarily by providers within a specific organization or clinic setting and contains internal information used by these organizational providers. Information within the EMR must be specifically sent to care providers who serve patients within organizations who have EHRs, and vice versa, as these systems do not spontaneously electronically exchange data and information.

TABLE 2.1 Difference Between EHR and EMR

Electronic Health Record (EHR)	Electronic Medical Record (EMR)
Digital record of total patient health history information from various clinicians and health care facilities	Digital version of patient chart of care provided within a health care facility
Offers patient portal for access to self-records and provider communication.	No patient portal feature for self-record retrieval or communication
Access to various tools used by health care providers for decision-making	Data used for provider patient diagnosis and treatment
Promotes sharing of real-time, up-to-date patient information through optimized transferability of data between organizations	Data not designed to be shared outside an organization or individual practice, which results in limited transferability of patient data between organizations

Personal Health Record

A **personal health record (PHR)** is an individual collection of medical documentation maintained by the person themselves or their authorized individual. This application generally includes the following:

- demographic data
- medical history with medical and surgical interventions
- allergies
- immunizations
- medications (past and present)
- diagnoses
- insurance information
- health providers contact information
- emergency contact information

Patients can add any other significant information they feel is important to include in their record. This includes self-reported and self-recorded information. These sources of information may include data from individual vital sign records or activity logs as well as data from personal devices such as smartphones and smart watches. Diet and nutrition management of medical conditions such as diabetes, obesity, cardiovascular disease, and so forth, may be added to this record. These records may be individually maintained in software packages, or some applications allow integration into the EMR.

The purpose of the PHR is to allow the patient to take control of their health care. This promotes active participation in personal health care management. This can enhance patient adherence and goal achievement for such medical conditions as hypertension and diabetes, for example. This will allow the patient to actively engage with care providers for identification of improvements or worsening of medical conditions for early intervention and potential problem resolution.

With benefits come potential weaknesses. Some of these weaknesses can include personal anxiety over one's conditions and obsessions regarding reporting data. This can result in over-recording of data and entry of numerous irrelevant data points. There can also be bias in reported data, with people only recording results that show compliance to medicines or regimens where none exists, if actual data were entered. There can also be security and confidentiality concerns with cloud-based data.

Overall, PHRs can have significant benefits, if used correctly. It has the potential to improve patient adherence, promote achievement of therapeutic goals, and conclude in achievement of collaborative patient/provider management of health care issues.

Chapter Summary

The EHR goes back to the 1960s when health care organizations started exploring computer-based methods of managing patient information. EHR evolution has progressed over decades due to technological advances, regulatory initiatives, and health care reform. Key milestones include HIPAA, HITECH, and the Privacy Rule. These, among others, served to shape EHR systems. Differentiating between the EHR and EMR, EHRs include a broader scope of patient information across various clinicians and several health care entities, whereas the EMR primarily focuses on clinical documentation within a single organization. PHRs promote active engagement in one's health care, allowing patients to track their metrics and make informed decisions about their care. As health care continues to evolve, these components will also change to further enhance care delivery, improve patient outcomes, and promote further health care policy. It is important for the EHR specialist to be an active participant in this development.

3

HEALTH CARE SYSTEMS

CHAPTER OBJECTIVES

Upon completion of this chapter, the reader will be able to do the following:

1. Describe the health care delivery system triad.
2. Differentiate between the Beveridge model, the Bismarck model, the National Health care model, and the Out-of-Pocket model of health care.
3. Define distinct types of delivery systems emerging in the United States.
4. Distinguish between various health care delivery models in the United States.

KEY CHAPTER TERMS

- Equity, cost, efficiency healthcare triad
- Beveridge model
- Bismarck model
- National Health care model
- Out-of-Pocket model
- Managed care
- Concierge services
- Self-directed services
- Telemedicine
- Health care delivery models and plans

Health Care Delivery Systems

The aim of systems used by governments and organizations is focused on the **equity, cost, and efficiency healthcare triad** (see Figure 3.1). Insurers and providers work within these health care delivery systems to promote all three components and deliver the best care possible.

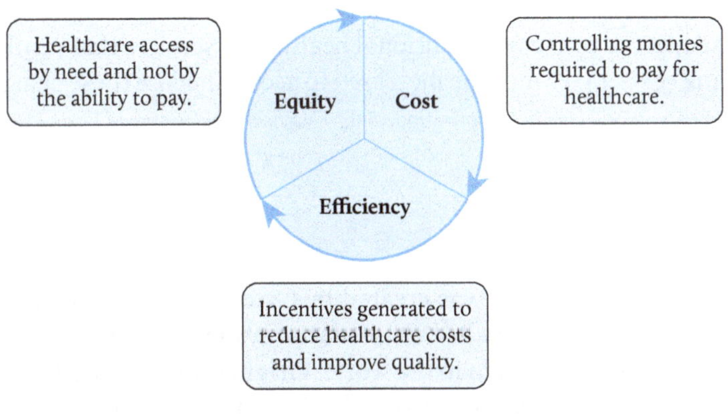

FIGURE 3.1 Triad of equity, cost and efficiency.

Reference: Bevin, G., Helderman, J., & Wilsford, D. (2010). Changing choices in health care: Implications for equity, efficiency and cost. *Health Economics, Policy and Law*, 5, 251–267.

Four Types of Health Care Models

Health care has been designed from four major models dating back as far as the 1800s and forms the foundation for care delivery worldwide. These models differ in funding and health care delivery structure. The United States uses all four of these models for various segments of its care delivery.

The Beveridge Model

The **Beveridge model** was created by Sir William Beveridge in 1948. There is a single payer in this system—the government. This system of health care is based on the principle of universal health care and funded by direct income tax deductions; thus, health care is free for patients. The universal health care system principle means that everyone is entitled to the full range of quality health care services (promotion to prevention, treatment, rehabilitation, and palliative care) when and where they need it regardless of their ability to pay (World Health Organization, n.d.).

One criticism of this system is overuse. Since there are no restrictions and access to health care is free, some patients demand services that are unnecessary, which promotes waste. Since this model is tax based, in order to cover additional health care services that result in rising costs, taxes must be increased to accommodate these charges.

Reference: World Health Organization. (n.d.). *Universal health coverage*. https://www.who.int/health-topics/universal-health-coverage#tab=tab_1

The Bismarck Model

The **Bismarck model** was created by Otto von Bismarck in 1883. This German statutory health insurance system was the first social health insurance system in the world. Originally developed to cover employed workers, it was expanded to include unemployed workers, non-earning wives and daughters, all primary dependents, and retirees by 1941. By 1981 students, artists, disabled persons, and farmers were covered under this system. Individuals who were self-employed and those who had earnings that exceeded the statutory health insurance threshold had an option for statutory insurance on a voluntary basis (Busse et al., 2017).

With the increase in German individual coverage came an increase in the scope and scale of benefits. This was both a benefit and disadvantage in the system. Beneficially, it improved care structures and improved patient services (e.g., inclusion of preventive health care check-ups and pediatric screenings). One big disadvantage was that it increased expenditures for health care overall as financial benefits improved (e.g., inclusion of 6 weeks full salary when sick for blue-collar workers, which formerly only applied to white-collar workers; Busse et al., 2017).

The Bismarck model has expanded to be used in several countries from its German start. Insurers in this model are called sickness funds. These funds are usually jointly financed by employers and employees. Hospitals and physicians are usually private and do not make a profit in this model (Wallace, 2013). Tight governmental regulations allow for cost control in this single-payer model.

References:

Busse, R., Blümel, M., Knieps, F., & Barnighausen, T. (2017). Statutory health insurance in Germany: A health system shaped by 135 years of solidarity, self-governance, and competition. *The Lancet, 380*(10097), 882–897. https://doi.org/10.1016/S0140-6736(17)31280-1

Wallace, L. (2013). A view of health care around the world. *Annals of Family Medicine, 11*(1). https://doi.org/10.1370/afm.1484

The National Health Care Model

The **National Health care model** is also called the National Health Insurance model. This health care model has elements of both the Beveridge model, in that the government acts as the single payer, and the Bismarck model, as providers are private. All citizens pay into the insurance program, which is run by the government. This universal insurance model does not make a profit or deny claims.

Since it does not require claim approval, nor does it have a financial profit motive, it is simpler to navigate for care services by the potential patient, which is an advantage. One criticism of this system is that as a result of the no claim refusal component, individuals must wait for extended times for care and treatment. This could be a significant disadvantage for serious health issues or cause simple issues to extend care requirements by the time care is actually received (Vera Whole Health, 2020).

Reference: Vera Whole Health. (2020). *Global healthcare: 4 major national models and how they work.* https://www.verawholehealth.com/blog/global-healthcare-4-major-national-models-and-how-they-work

The Out-of-Pocket Model

The **Out-of-Pocket model** is generally thought of as monies paid by individuals for direct health care services without other forms of insurance or financial assistance. Technically, the out-of-pocket model for patient spending is part of all models, whether it be for full uninsured care requirements or as copayments for partial insurance reimbursement. Out-of-pocket can be conceptualized "as the sum of cost sharing requirements for covered or insured services, direct payments for uncovered/uninsured services, and informal payments" (Rice et al., 2018, p. 3).

The ability to pay has a direct effect on access to care. In countries where health care is based on income as little to no government assistance systems exist, persons who can afford to pay for health care receive care while those without the ability to pay (uninsured) either stay sick, get some disease relief by using home remedies, or die due to disease progression. Thus, those who can afford to pay for health care receive it and those without the ability to pay do not have access due to its financial burden. Health care financial burden can also result in bankruptcy and subsequent loss of care access and move individuals from one model to another.

Reference: Rice, T., Quentin, W., Anell, A., Barnes, A. J., Rosenau, P., Unruh, L. Y., & van Ginneken, E. (2018). Revisiting out-of-pocket requirements: Trends in spending, financial access barriers, and policy in ten high-income countries. *BMC Health Services Research*, *18*(1), 371. https://doi.org/10.1186/s12913-018-3185-8

Health Care Delivery Systems in the United States

Health care trends and varying types of delivery systems are emerging in the United States (see Table 3.1). These affect how individuals interact with the system they decide to use in their care delivery. This decision can be beneficial as the system often coordinates with one of the models used in the country and can enhance care received by patients.

TABLE 3.1 Health Care Delivery Systems

Classification	Information
Managed Care	• Overall aim is to control costs and improve care quality through coordination and management of health care services provided to a specific group of patients, often through a health care provider network. • Patients in the system generally belong to a health plan or insurance network in that their care is overseen by a primary care provider who is the gatekeeper for any specialty care. • Utilization management, case management, and disease management are used for appropriate cost-effective care delivery. • Managed Care includes the following: ◦ Health Maintenance Organizations (HMOs) that offer preventive care and other services for a monthly fee.

	◦ Preferred Provider Organizations (PPOs) that offer a fee-for-service system. ◦ Point-of-Service (POS) plans that allow for out-of-network referrals at a higher cost.
Concierge services	• Services also known as retainer-based or boutique medicine. • Patients pay an annual fee or retainer to a care provider for enhanced access to personalized and more comprehensive medical services. • Care providers often have smaller patient clientele load, which allows more time dedicated to patients who receive more direct and personalized care. • Services often provide same day appointments and 24/7 care provider access with more convenient coordination of care.
Self-directed services	• This is a consumer-driven health care service. • Individuals in the system have more control over their health care decisions. • Care and services are directed by the individual desiring care. • Consumers select their health care providers and treatments, determining where their health care dollars are spent. • Services may be paid for through the use of consumer health savings accounts (HSAs) or flexible spending accounts (FSAs).
Telemedicine	• Service provides remote delivery of information and medical services through telecommunications technology. • Services provided through video conferencing, telephone calls, or an online program for delivery of patient care by the health care provider. • The need for in-person care delivery, including assessment, diagnosis, and treatment, is reduced by this service. • Access to care for individuals who may have difficulty getting to an onsite office visit due to barriers, which may include physical disability and transportation, is increased through telecommunications technology.

Health Care Delivery Models in the United States

Health care delivery models and plans for obtaining care for the consumer can vary. These dictate the types of insurance coverage and how care can be accessed. These plans combine services and components from the identified models as well as the system types to offer a foundational component for care access by consumers and delivery by care providers (see Table 3.2).

TABLE 3.2 Consumer Models/Plans for Care

Plan Name	Abbreviation	Specifics
Health Maintenance Organization	HMO	• Primary care physician selected, and one must see this person first for illness or injury. • Advantage: Cost typically less than other insurance forms. • Disadvantage: Network restriction for care. Care outside network requires physician referral.
Preferred Provider Organization	PPO	• May have no requirement for primary care physician. Network of various providers provided for selection based on need. • Advantage: Greater flexibility for provider selection. Out of network care provided. • Disadvantage: Increased cost.
Point of Service	POS	• Hybrid plan between a PPO and HMO. Combining features of both. • Advantage: Greater care selection flexibility. • Disadvantage: Specialized care access requires physician referral.

Exclusive Provider Organization	EPO	• Includes characteristics of both an HMO and PPO. Does not require primary care physician. • Advantage: Access to specialized care without referral required. • Disadvantage: Network may restrict specialized care access.
Private Fee-for-Service	PFFS	• A specific consumer Medicare Advantage plan offered by various insurance companies. The company determines the level of cost sharing between patient and health care provider. No primary care physician nor referral required. • Advantage: Many do not have a network, so there is no restriction. • Disadvantage: Provider may or may not accept insurance offered plan, which can restrict care access.
Special Needs Plan	SNP	• A specific consumer Medicare Advantage plan that is for individuals with specific health needs or diseases. Provider list customized for specific care needs. Primary care physician or care coordinator required. A specialist referral is required for most plans. • Advantage: Specialized care provided to address specific health conditions. • Disadvantage: Not available in all states.

Chapter Summary

The health care system triad encompasses three key components, which include equity, cost, and efficiency. Equity relates to care access based on need; cost relates to the financial aspect for health care services; and incentives are set to ultimately improve care quality. Health care has been designed from four major models dating back as far as the 1800s. These include the Beveridge model, the Bismarck model, the National Health Insurance model, and the Out-of-Pocket model, which form the foundation for care delivery worldwide. These reflect different approaches to organizing and financing health care systems. The United States uses a combination of these to develop and implement consumer models and plans for its citizens care such as HMOs, PPOs, POSs, EPOs, PFFS, and SNPs. The EHRS uses this foundational and current information as it provides context within the broader health care landscape. It promotes strategic decision-making for organizational success.

4

HEALTH CARE SETTINGS AND PERSONNEL

CHAPTER OBJECTIVES

Upon completion of this chapter, the reader will be able to do the following:

1. Recognize key services for different health care settings.
2. Summarize various health care settings for care delivery.
3. Define a *health care professional*.
4. Differentiate various health care professional roles.

KEY CHAPTER TERMS

- Hospitals/Medical centers
- Clinics
- Urgent care centers
- Rehabilitation centers
- Home health care
- Hospice care
- Physicians
- Nurses
- Physician Assistants
- Pharmacists
- Respiratory therapists
- Physical therapists
- Occupational therapists
- Clinical social workers

Health Care Settings

There are many settings where health care is delivered. Patients receive a broad range of health care services, from small clinics to large medical and trauma centers.

Hospitals/Medical Centers

Hospitals and medical centers offer full medical care, which includes diagnostic services to interventional inpatient and outpatient services. Diagnostic services include radiological specialty services such as scans and imaging. Inpatient services include all services required to improve the health of an individual who requires onsite care. These patients stay overnight and may stay for days to weeks based on the severity of their illness. Outpatient services include those services inclusive of surgical intervention where an individual can be treated and following the procedure sent to a post-anesthesia care area to wake up and then be sent home for full recovery and further follow-up care by friends and family. They do not remain overnight following an outpatient surgical procedure.

Clinics

Clinics are smaller than hospital and medical centers and are where routine preventative care can be administered to individuals. They provide general primary care services (wellness examinations, vaccinations, non-emergency care) to specialized services (women's health, pediatrics, mental health). These patients are usually less sick and do not require overnight health care activities or interventions.

Urgent Care Centers

Urgent care centers provide care for illnesses, injuries, or conditions that require prompt attention but are not life-threatening or so serious that they require emergency room intervention (e.g., can provide X-ray for a sprained ankle with significant swelling to identify if there are other injuries). These centers are often open during and after regular clinic hours, which makes them easily accessible for the daytime working individual. They are not intended to replace but supplement care by a primary provider as they focus on treatment of short-term health care issues and not chronic illnesses that require long-term medication regimens and continuous treatment.

Rehabilitation Centers

Rehabilitation centers provide care for individuals recovering from an injury, illness, or surgery and are not able to take care of themselves at home. These centers provide 24-hour care and services to help a person regain their strength and mobility. This allows a return to the ability to perform activities of daily living for self-care (e.g., dressing oneself, walking, cooking, brushing one's teeth, taking a bath or shower, etc.). Rehabilitation services may be promoted by non-rehabilitation centers by changing the patient's service status to swing bed or by transferring the actual patient to a skilled nursing facility wing within the existing inpatient facility.

Home Health Care

Home health care is care provided in one's home. A care provider (nurse or aide) comes to the home to conveniently administer needed care. This care is aimed at promoting a return to independence and preventing condition decline. It can also provide care for components needed for other health care activities such as special types of intravenous lines for nutrition, activities of daily living and therapies, or cancer medication administration.

Hospice Care

Hospice care provides end-of-life care. It focuses on care and comfort to promote quality of life for a dying person who is seriously ill. The purpose of this care is no longer curative but to offer physical, emotional, social, and spiritual support for the patient and their family members as the patient approaches the end of their life. The goal of this care is to manage pain and promote comfort. It can be given at home or in an extended care facility, nursing home, or hospital.

The EHR for these health care settings will be specific to activities performed as well as insurance requirements and best care practice requirements. Privacy and security standards will facilitate retrieval and storage of these required patient data components, as approved on the forms and templates.

Health Care Personnel

A health care professional is an individual with earned credentials who is licensed, registered, or certified based on requirements set by the federal government or state laws or regulations to provide health care services to healthy or ill patients. They have been educated and demonstrated acquired knowledge in general and specific areas of care delivery. They work together and with other providers to deliver the best care possible to patients. You may see these category abbreviations in charts or after the first initial and last name of the provider in the chart.

Physicians

The **physician's** category of health care individuals includes medical doctors (MDs) and Doctor of Osteopathic Medicine (DO-focus on providing holistic practices, which include treating the whole person for preventative health and healing). Physicians may be a generalist (family practice physician) or a specialist (neurologist [focuses on nervous problems and disorders], gynecologist [focuses on women's health], cardiologist [focuses on problems and disorders of the heart], nephrologist [focuses on problems and diseases of the kidneys], etc.).

Nurses

The **nurse's** category of health care individuals includes registered nurses (RNs), licensed practical nurses (LPNs), licensed vocational nurses (LVNs), and advanced practice registered nurses (APRNs). RNs are individuals who graduated from a nursing program (generally 2 or 4 years) and passed a state-based licensure examination. They provide care in all health care settings. LPNs are individuals with a high school diploma or GED, who have graduated from an approved program (generally 1 to 2 years) and are licensed by the state as a caregiver. These individuals deliver care in all areas of health care under the supervision of an RN. LVNs are individuals with a high school completion or GED who have attended an educational program and graduated with a certificate in less than 2 years. This position focuses on clinical aspects of patient care under the direct supervision of an RN. The APRN is an individual who has received education beyond the basic college education (a master's degree [Master of Science in Nursing, MSN] or Doctor of Nursing Practice [DNP] degree). They are often referred to as mid-level providers. The APRN may be educated in a special area of care delivery such as a Nurse Practitioner (NP; may be in a specialized practitioner area such as a Family Nurse Practitioner [FNP], Acute Care Nurse Practitioner [ACNP], Pediatric Nurse Practitioner [PNP], etc.), Certified Nurse Midwife (CNM), or Clinical Nurse Specialist (CNS). APRNs can diagnose and treat (including prescribing) individuals independent of a physician. They may own and manage their own independent practice or clinic. Nurses work in all areas of health care.

Physician Assistants

Being a **Physician Assistant** (PA) requires a bachelor's degree for entry and additional master's-level educational training over a 24- to 27-month period. They are often referred to as mid-level providers and may require a health care background for program entry. The PA may diagnose and treat under the direct supervision of a physician. According to the American Academy of Physician Assistants (2019), the PA role is based on "education and experience; state law; policies of employers and facilities, and the needs of the patients" (para. 1).

Reference: American Academy of Physician Assistants. (2019, September). *PA scope of practice.* https://www.aapa.org/wp-content/uploads/2017/01/Issue-brief_Scope-of-Practice_0117-1.pdf

Pharmacists

Pharmacists are focused on medicinal intervention for patients in both inpatient and outpatient settings. Practicing individuals may be a Registered Pharmacist (RPh) (a 5-year degree possible to be earned prior to 2000) or have a Doctor of Pharmacy (PharmD) degree (currently the standard 6-year degree). Both have passed licensure requirements to practice as a pharmacist. They ensure that medications are safely prescribed and dispensed. They also make sure that patients have the proper education to safely take their prescribed medications and know side effects. The RPh and PharmD knowledge base allows them to identify potential problems, resolve problems that have occurred, and prevent drug-related problems through drug reconciliation (review of all medications, including those over the counter [OTC] or not prescribed and herbs taken by the patient).

Respiratory Therapists

Respiratory therapists manage patients with respiratory (breathing) and cardiopulmonary disorders. Certification for this area of health care includes the certified respiratory therapist (CRT) and registered respiratory therapist (RRT) certifications. The individual with a CRT credential completes an accredited respiratory therapy program of study with a minimum of an associate degree and successfully passes a credentialing examination. An individual with the RRT credential either has an associate, bachelor's, or master's degree in respiratory therapy. Individuals with these credentials evaluate, treat, and care for patients in various settings, including hospitals, clinics rehabilitation centers, and even in patient homes. They work to improve respiration and oxygen exchange by performing breathing treatments, giving oxygen therapy, giving aerosol treatments, managing mechanical ventilation, and breathing for the patient during cardiopulmonary resuscitation.

Physical Therapists

Physical therapists (PTs) are licensed professionals who specialize in restoring mobility, reducing pain, and improving patient quality of health. The PT works with individuals who have injuries or health conditions that result in reduced mobility or limitations in movement to such a degree that it interferes with their ability to provide for their own self-care (e.g., arthritis that reduces patient ability to perform activities of daily living, knee surgery, hip surgery, sports injuries, motor vehicle accidents, motorcycle accidents, etc.).

Occupational Therapists

Occupational therapists (OTs) are focused on improving a patient's ability to perform daily activities and tasks that allow them to be independent and possibly return to being a productive individual in the work force. The OT works to evaluate and treat patients with illnesses, injuries, or disabilities, to help them in various settings which include hospitals, clinics, and homes. The goal of their patient intervention outcome is promotion of independence.

Clinical Social Workers

Clinical Social Workers (CSWs) are focused on counseling and support for patients and families as they deal with social issues as well as mental health issues. These individuals assess, diagnose, and treat patients and families to promote prevention of mental, emotional, and other behavioral problems. The CSW is licensed or certified in their state of practice. The CSW works in various settings, which include primary care offices, hospitals, mental health clinics, and community agencies.

Training, education, and certifications can vary by state. These validate expertise and qualifications in the specific area of specialization. This is not a comprehensive list but an example of just a few of the many diverse types of health care professionals in various health care settings. In addition, as care evolves there will be others added to the list of care providers, both for specialization and primary care delivery.

Chapter Summary

Understanding key services across various health care settings is essential for the EHRS. Health care settings vary widely, ranging from hospitals to clinics, to long-term care, with each serving different primary patient populations. Each of these settings offer distinct services to address unique patient needs. Health care professionals play critical roles in delivering care across these settings. They provide medical treatment, preventive services, and therapeutic interventions. There is a diverse range of roles within health care inclusive of physicians, nurses, pharmacists, and so forth. Each role performs responsibilities within their scope of practice that contribute to collaborative patient management. When the EHRS can differentiate settings and understand professional roles, they can ensure accurate data management.

5

LAWS AND REGULATIONS GOVERNING EHRS

CHAPTER OBJECTIVES

Upon completion of this chapter, the reader will be able to do the following:

1. Interpret HIPAA.
2. Interpret the HITECH Act.
3. Discuss the Medicare and CHIP (Children's Health Insurance Program) Reauthorization Act (MACRA).
4. Differentiate regulations and guidelines that govern claims submission and reimbursement.
5. Define *Meaningful Use* and its transition to the Medicare Promoting Interoperability Program.
6. Explain the 21st Century Cures Act.

KEY CHAPTER TERMS

- HIPAA
- HITECH Act
- Medicare Access and CHIP (Children's Health Insurance Program) Reauthorization Act (MACRA)
- Merit-Based Incentive Payment System (MIPS)
- Alternative Payment Models (APMs)
- Meaningful Use
- Medicare Promoting Interoperability Program
- U.S. Food and Drug Administration (FDA)
- International Classification of Diseases (ICD) codes

- National Correct Coding Initiative (NCCI)
- Current Procedural Terminology (CPT) codes
- Electronic Data Interchange (EDI) standards
- Institute of Electrical and Electronics Engineers (IEEE)
- The 21st Century Cures Act (Cures Act)

Laws and Regulations

The EHR has been shown to improve patient outcomes, but it is also subject to various laws and regulations. These are designed to keep records safe and ensure patient access. All health care providers and organizations that provide health services that use the EHR for patient record keeping must comply with these laws and regulations.

HIPAA

Prior to **HIPAA**, the Privacy Act of 1974 was created to address concerns about the creation and use of computerized databases and how these might affect individual privacy rights. This precursor to HIPAA was created to address concerns regarding how the creation and use of computerized databases might affect the privacy rights of patients. This goal was achieved by restricting disclosure of personally identifiable information; granting persons increased access rights to agency records; granting an individual the right to amend agency records by supplying proof that the maintained record is not accurate, relevant, timely, or complete; and establishing a code of fair information practices.

In the early 1990s, health care was undergoing a technology boom, which resulted in organizations using more computerized systems to collect payment for claims, collect eligibility information, and many other administrative actions related to patient health care data. The Health Insurance Portability and Accountability Act (HIPAA) was passed in 1996 and required the U.S. Department of Health and Human Services (HHS) to provide regulations to protect the privacy and security of patient personal health information. Prior to HIPAA there were no generally accepted security standards or general requirements to protect health information. Two documents were developed and published to address the HHS requirement. One addressed privacy, the HIPAA Privacy Rule, and the other security, the HIPAA Security Rule. The HIPAA Privacy Rule establishes national standards to protect medical records and other identifiable health information, which is collectively known as "protected health information". The HIPAA Privacy Rule sets limits and conditions on uses and disclosures of protected health information without a person's authorization. This rule gives patients the right to examine their own records, request corrections, and obtain a copy of these records. Patients also must give permission for their records to be sent to a third party. The HIPAA Security Rule establishes national standards to protect electronic personal information that is created, received, used, or maintained by entities with permission to have them. This rule requires safeguards (administrative, physical, and technical) to ensure confidentiality, integrity, and security of electronic protected health information (ePHI) but is flexible and scalable to allow growth of organizational systems. This growth results from technologies that are appropriate to facilitate structural expansion of an organization, which may be necessary to improve patient outcomes.

Compliance with the Privacy and Security Rule is mandatory, and enforcement falls under the responsibility of the Office of Civil Rights (OCR). The OCR uses the HIPAA Enforcement Rule, which outlines procedures for investigating and enforcing violations. Financial penalties are levied against organizations that do not comply with these rules. No state law can exempt an organization from complying with any of these rules. Federal requirements preempt state law, which means that the federal law supersedes any state law related to HIPAA. The HIPAA breach notification rule requires HIPAA-covered organizations to provide notification following unauthorized access or potential access and retrieval of protected health information. This means that security and privacy of health information has been compromised and individuals with no right to an ePHI have retrieved it through an unauthorized intrusion into the electronic system that houses this information for an organization whether on premises or in the cloud.

HIPAA can be challenging, but in order to ensure organization compliance with rules, knowledge of this act and all its components is mandatory. The Department of Health and Human Services has several sites to assist with identification of key rule components. The one for health care professionals is located at https://www.hhs.gov/hipaa/for-professionals/index.html.

HITECH Act

The **HITECH Act** was initiated in 2009 to provide financial incentives ranging from as much as $18,000 in year 1 to a reduction to $2,000 by year 5 to health care providers and organizations to promote adoption of a certified electronic health record system. The program was to ensure meaningful use of these systems and identify penalties for those who failed to comply with HITECH regulations. This federal program was part of the American Recovery and Reinvestment Act (ARRA).

The goal of HITECH was to promote widespread EHR and other health information technology (HIT) adoption. EHR promotion was intended to improve health care quality and efficiency, reduce health care costs, and improve patient outcomes. HITECH provided financial incentives for reaching specified milestones by specific dates for EHR implementation by a health care provider. The provider had to verify adoption and demonstrate meaningful use of a certified EHR technology to be eligible for incentive payments.

HITECH also included privacy and security provisions. These strengthened HIPAA regulation enforcement, increased penalties for HIPAA noncompliance, and identified new breach notification requirements.

Medicare Access and CHIP Reauthorization Act

What is CHIP (Children's Health Insurance Program) you might ask? CHIP makes funds available for states to provide health care coverage for low-income uninsured children through the age of 18 years and pregnant women who have an income too high to qualify for Medicaid. The **Medicare Access and CHIP Reauthorization Act** (MACRA), which was a federal law enacted in 2015, included this in its reauthorization act. MACRA replaced the Sustainable Growth Rate (SGR) formula for physician payment, which reformed the Medicare payment model and encouraged a shift to value-based care. The SGR used a formula for physician payment based on growth of the economy and not quality or access to care. The new payment model rewarded health care providers for the delivery of high-quality, cost-effective care over the volume of care provided.

MACRA set up two pathways under the Quality Payment Program (QPP), the **Merit-Based Incentive Payment System (MIPS)** and **Alternative Payment Models (APMs)**. Providers will select one of these pathways, which will link their payments to the quality of care provided.

MIPS is a performance-based payment system with five health care participation options:

- Individual: The health care provider submits their own individual data.
- Group: The health care provider practice or group submits data on behalf of all participating clinicians under one tax identification number.
- Virtual group: Two or more tax identification numbers that elect to form a collective group for a performance year.
- Subgroup: A subset of health care providers (two or more) that has at least one individual MIPS-eligible clinician.
- APM entity: A MIPS eligible group or individual who participates in the MIPS APM who is collectively approved to submit data as an aggregate across multiple tax identification numbers.

MIPS uses four performance categories to measure care quality. MACRA adjusts Medicare payment rates to providers based on scores earned in these categories.

- Quality: Clinical quality performance is determined by specific measures, which include patient outcomes, safety, and the patient experience (patient satisfaction), which is compared to preidentified benchmarks.
- Interoperability promotion: Use of the EHR to exchange health information with other providers and patients is evaluated. This category requires providers to report on measures used to promote patient engagement, exchange of health information, and other specific activities that promote EHR use that improve patient care.
- Improvement activities: Health care providers report on improvement activities they have implemented that are selected from a list of options provided by the Center for Medicare and Medicaid (CMS).
- Care cost: Providers are evaluated on the cost of care they provide to patients. This is a cost calculation based on Medicare claims data.

APMs are a pathway that encourage health care providers to focus on innovative payment approaches rather than fee-for-service payment models. It is designed to encourage providers to deliver high-quality care more efficiently using incentives. Key elements include the following:

- Providers are rewarded for achieving cost savings and meeting quality benchmarks.
- A variety of payment models are encouraged which include Accountable Care Organizations (ACOs) and bundled payments.
- The pathway operates on a two-track system.
  - An Advanced APM system has providers who meet specific criteria and are willing to accept a certain level of financial risk can qualify. They may be exempt from MIPS reporting and be eligible for additional incentives.
  - A second 'other' APM system has providers who are designated as Qualifying APR Participants (QPs). These providers do not qualify as Advanced APMs but may qualify for APM status if they meet certain patient and payment thresholds. QPs may be exempt from MIPS reporting and be eligible for additional bonuses.

CMS set the performance threshold to 100: quality 30%, cost 30%, promoting interoperability 25%, and improvement activities 15%. The final score is determined based on overall performance. This determines payment adjustment percentages. The 2023 threshold was set to 75 points, with payment adjustments ranging from -9% to +9%. If the final score is below the threshold, the health care provider will receive a negative adjustment to Medicare Part B payments. If the final score is equal to the threshold, the health care provider will not receive any payment adjustments. If the final score is above the threshold the health care provider will receive a positive adjustment (Physicians Advocacy Institute, 2023).

Reference: Physicians Advocacy Institute. (2023). *2023 Merit-Based Incentive Payment System (MIPS) scoring overview.* http://www.physiciansadvocacyinstitute.org/Portals/0/assets/docs/MIPS-Pathway/MIPS%20Scoring%20Overview.pdf

Meaningful Use

Meaningful use refers to the use of certified EHR technology by health care providers to specifically improve the safety, efficiency, and quality of patient care. CMS introduced the meaningful use concept in 2011 as part of the Medicare and Medicaid EHR incentive programs to encourage the widespread adoption of the EHR by health care providers and organizations in the United States. CMS offered incentives for the use of certified EHR technology. Meaningful use set specific guidelines that eligible professionals and organizations had to achieve in order to participate in the EHR incentive program. There were three stages of Meaningful use that extended from 2011 through 2016 (see Figure 5.1).

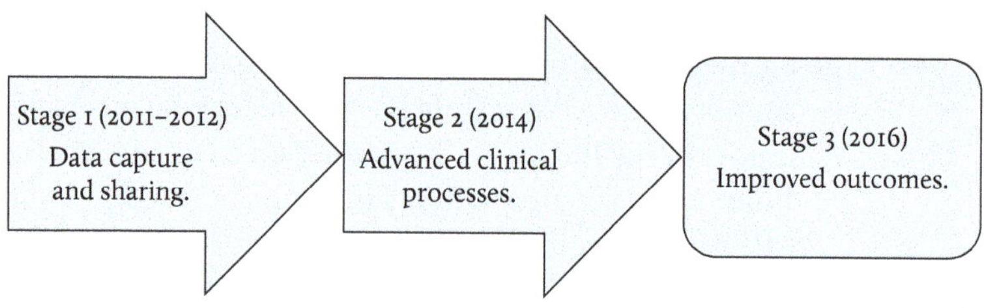

FIGURE 5.1 Three stages of Meaningful Use.

Criteria for each stage increased in complexity and requirements. Some requirements included the following:

- use of computerized physician order entry (CPOE) for patient medication orders
- implementation of an electronic component for identification of drug-to-drug and drug allergy interactions
- implementation and use of support tools for clinical decision-making
- use of the ability to exchange patient health information with other care providers for patients
- list generation of patients with specific conditions for promotion of quality improvement purposes

Health care providers had to demonstrate meaningful use through an attestation process based on the timeline for each meaningful use reporting period. This required that eligible professionals successfully (a) use a certified EHR system; (b) meet meaningful objectives (20 of 25), core objectives (15 of the 20 meaningful objectives) and menu set objectives (5 of 10); and (c) report clinical quality measures. Failure to participate in meaningful use resulted in a penalty (reduced Medicare reimbursements; Anumula & Sanelli, 2012).

Reference: Anumula, N., & Sanelli, P. C. (2012). Meaningful Use. *AJNR: American Journal of Neuroradiology*, *33*(8), 1455–1457. https://doi.org/10.3174/ajnr.A3247

Meaningful Use leveraged EHR technology to achieve the best outcomes for patients, which included the following:

- quality of care improvement
- improved patient safety
- reduced health disparities
- patient and family engagement
- improved care coordination
- improved overall public health
- maintenance of patient information privacy and security

Meaningful Use ultimately aimed to improve population health, empower individuals, increase information transparency, and improve and increase research data retrieval.

Physicians and care providers who did not participate in Meaningful Use received a penalty in the form of reduced Medicare reimbursements for care delivery. Physicians and other providers were required to use certified electronic health records and demonstrate meaningful use. At the end of each reporting period care providers were required to submit an attestation process to avoid receiving a penalty.

The Meaningful Use program moved beyond the existing requirements in 2018, becoming known as the Medicare and **Medicaid Promoting Interoperability Program**. In 2022 there was an additional change with the discontinuation of the Medicaid Promoting Interoperability Program. This left the Medicare Promoting Interoperability Program active. These name changes came with some programmatic final changes in 2023 as well, which included mandatory reporting on the four objectives of electronic prescribing, health information exchange, provider-to-patient exchange, and public health and clinical data exchange. Ultimately organizations now must demonstrate their use of the EHR that can be measured against these identified standards. As technology continues to progress, there will undoubtedly be future updates and changes.

MERIT-BASED INCENTIVE PAYMENT SYSTEM: A MEANINGFUL USE REPLACEMENT

Meaningful Use was incorporated as part of the MIPS. It was transitioned into this program to be one of the components of the Merit-Based Payment System (MIPS). The MIPS includes the Physician Quality Reporting Program (PQRS), Value-Based Payment Modifier (VM), and Merit EHR Incentive program also known as Meaningful Use. The MIPS is also part of the Medicare Access and CHIP Reauthorization Act (MACRA), which was enacted in 2015 by the U.S. Congress but officially began January 1, 2017. MIPS was designed to streamline existing Medicare incentive programs that were perceived as burdensome and complex to navigate and implement. Through consolidation, it incorporated several existing programs to simplify reporting and incentive process for the Physician Quality Reporting System (PQRS), the Value-Based Payment Modifier (VM), and the Medicare Electronic Health Record (EHR) Incentive Program (Meaningful Use).

The intention of MACRA is to transition how Medicare pays. It promotes payment for value-based care instead of fee-for-service. Eligible clinicians under MIPS include physicians, nurse practitioners and physician assistants. Each are addressed below:

> *Physician*: A physician is a medical doctor (MD), Doctor of Osteopathic Medicine (DO; focuses on the whole-body approach to care), Doctor of Dental Surgery (DDS), Doctor of Dentistry or Dental Medicine (DMD), Doctor of Podiatric Medicine (DPM; focuses on diagnosing and treating conditions of the foot, ankle, and leg structures), and Doctor of Optometry (OD; focuses on examining, diagnosing, treating, and managing eye diseases). All are eligible under MIPS. They are licensed medical professionals who assess, diagnose, and treat patient illnesses and injuries. These individuals complete a bachelor's degree, medical school education, and a residency in a specialty of medicine. They can prescribe medications; order diagnostic tests; perform medical procedures, including surgeries, if this is within their scope of practice and within their specialty; and provide focused or comprehensive/total patient care.

Chiropractor: Chiropractors do not hold a MD degree, so they are not known as medical doctors, but they have received the Doctor of Chiropractic (DC) degree. These individuals complete a bachelor's degree and a 4-year chiropractic education prior to licensure. If they choose to specialize, they may extend their education and residency by 2 to 3 years. They have received training in using their hands to manipulate body parts to address various conditions as well as for pain relief. Most do not prescribe drugs but focus on prescribing solutions that do not require drugs, such as massage therapy, physical therapy, heat/ice therapy, and so on. These services and treatments complement chiropractic care.

Advanced Practice Registered Nurse (APRN): An APRN is an individual with specialization with a minimum of an advanced degree in nursing (master's or doctorate). These include Nurse Practitioners (NPs), Clinical Nurse Specialists (CNSs), Certified Registered Nurse Anesthetists (CRNAs) and Certified Nurse Midwives. These individuals have specialized education to perform care within their scope of practice. The NP and CNS are licensed nursing professionals who assess, diagnose, and treat various patient illnesses and injuries. The CRNA works directly with patients delivering anesthesia during surgery and procedures. The Nurse Midwife works with patients throughout their pregnancy and can facilitate delivery in various settings. They can prescribe medications, order diagnostic tests, perform medical procedures based on their area of specialty (e.g., acute care, family nursing, nurse anesthetist, women's health, nurse midwife, geriatric women's health, etc.) and provide comprehensive or total patient care. The APRN collaborates with physicians and other health care professionals.

Physician Assistant: A Physician Assistant (PA) is a certified health care professional. They are trained to provide a range of medical services. They can perform physical examinations, diagnose, and treat certain illnesses; order and interpret diagnostic tests; and prescribe some medications based on their specific training background. The PA typically completes an undergraduate and master's degree program of specific study. The PA may work in a hospital, clinic, or physician office and works under the supervision of a licensed physician.

Therapist: Physical and Occupational therapists focus on improving functional ability. These individuals complete a bachelor's degree and graduate education prior to certification and licensure. The Occupational Therapist is currently required to hold a minimum of a Master of Occupational Therapy (MOT) degree, but some individuals obtain a Doctor of Occupational Therapy (OTD) degree. The Physical Therapist is required to hold a Doctor of Physical Therapy (DPT) degree to practice. The Physical Therapist focuses on improving a patient's mobility following a medical incident (e.g., stroke), accidental injury, or surgical intervention. The Occupational Therapist focuses on a patient's ability to perform activities of daily living for better functioning. Both of these rehabilitative therapists improve a patient's ability for independent living and overall quality of life.

Qualified Speech-Language Pathologist (SLP): An SLP focuses on improving speech and addressing swallowing issues. These individuals complete a bachelor's degree in a health-related field and generally 2 years of postbaccalaureate study for a master's degree along with a supervised clinical experience or fellowship. Licensure is a requirement in all states, and certification can serve to address additional state requirements. The SLP is educated to assess, diagnose, and treat speech, language, social and cognitive communication, and swallowing disorders in children and adults. This includes voice and fluency disorders. Addressing these disorders is essential to promoting a patient being verbally understood by others so that they can create meaningful relationships.

Qualified Audiologist: An audiologist must earn a doctoral degree in the field in order to be licensed and certified. This generally requires 4 years of undergraduate education and 4 or more years in a Doctor of Audiology (AuD), Doctor of Philosophy (PhD), or combined AuD/PhD program of study. They complete an externship year of study before taking the licensure examination and certification. The audiologist is educated to assess, diagnose, treat, manage, as well as prevent hearing loss and balance disorders in persons of all ages. This promotes better balance and an improved quality of life through the ability to hear sounds for safety and pleasure.

Registered Dieticians or Nutrition Professionals: A Registered Dietician (RD) is a board-certified individual who is an expert in food and nutrition, human nutrition, dietetics, or food systems. These individuals earn at a minimum a bachelor's degree, and some individuals complete graduate study (master's). Both degrees are followed by an internship. Following education and internship one can qualify for the RD board examination. Some states require licensure to practice. The RD is knowledgeable regarding nutrition and dietetics and their impact on health. They manage nutrition for acute and chronic conditions. Nutrition Professionals may or may not have a specific educational foundation based on their state of practice. They offer more general nutritional advice and cannot offer medical treatment related to nutrition.

Clinical Social Worker: The Clinical Social Worker (CSW) is an individual who focuses on mental and emotional illnesses. They have earned a bachelor's degree in social work. A person licensed at this educational level can provide nonclinical social work (e.g., management, mediation, etc.). In order to practice as a CSW, a graduate degree (master's) is required, with an additional 2 years of supervised work in the field. Licensure is required to use the title Social Worker in many states. They assess, diagnose, treat, and work to provide mental health services and address behavioral and biopsychological problems and disorders.

These MIPS-eligible care providers are evaluated on four performance categories:

1. Quality: This category assesses care quality provided by eligible clinicians based on a variety of performance measures. These reported quality measures are compared to benchmarks for a score calculation. Measures cover a range of clinical areas, which include preventive care, management of chronic diseases, and patient safety. Quality accounts for 45% of the MIPS composite score.
2. Cost: This category evaluates eligible cost of clinician-provided care on Medicare claims data. CMS uses claims data to calculate this area, so no additional provider report is required. Cost accounts for 15% of the MIPS composite score.
3. Improvement activities: This category measures activities that aim to improve clinical practice and patient care for eligible care provider clinicians. Clinicians select from a list of improvement activities provided by CMS and generate a report. Activities focus on specific areas that include care coordination, patient engagement, and population health management. Improvement activities account for 15% of the MIPS composite score.
4. Promoting Interoperability (PI): This category was formerly known as Advancing Care Information (ACI). It assesses eligible clinician EHR use and their ability to electronically exchange patient health information. Reported measures in this category relate to electronic prescribing, health information exchange, patient access to health information, and other functionalities of an EHR. Promoting interoperability activity accounts for 25% of the MIPS composite score.

The MIPS program aims to serve as an incentive to the promotion of high-quality, cost-efficient care practices and the meaningful use of health information technology by providers. The clinician or care provider's total composite score is compared to a performance threshold set by CMS. Based on their level above or below the threshold, payment adjustment is made. Those providers above the threshold may receive a positive payment adjustment, while those below the set threshold may receive a negative payment adjustment to their Medicare Part B payments. The intent of the MIPS program is to serve as an incentive to improve care processes and health outcomes, increase health care information use, and reduce care costs.

APMS: A MEANINGFUL USE REPLACEMENT

Advanced Alternative Payment Models (APMs) were enacted in 2015. They are part of the Medicare Access and CHIP Reauthorization Act (MACRA). Their aim is to reform the way Medicare pays health care providers and promote a transition from fee-for-service to value-based care. APMs are one of two payment tracks under MACRA. The other MACRA payment track is MIPS.

APMs are intended to add an incentive component for health care providers to participate in models that may involve more financial risk for patient care quality and cost of care. These models hold care providers accountable for patient health outcomes. High-quality care that results in better outcomes is rewarded monetarily. Care providers must meet qualifications set by CMS, which include participation in the Medicare Shared Savings Program (MSSP).

Care providers who participate in Advanced APMs can earn a 5% payment on their Medicare Part B payments, starting in 2019 through 2024. If these providers meet certain thresholds, they are exempt from participating in MIPS and reporting under MIPS. Advanced APMs are thought to play a significant role in promoting changes in health care and transforming the health care system toward a value-based system. It is designed to emphasize improvement in patient outcomes and reduce unnecessary health care cost for patients in the United States.

U.S. Food and Drug Administration Regulations

EHRs are currently not regulated by the **U.S. Food and Drug Administration (FDA)**, but they have issued guidance on EHR use in clinical trials and provided recommendations for safety and usability improvements. The FDA does accept data for clinical trials for decision-making purposes, but they must be able to verify data integrity and quality during inspections.

The FDA established the Digital Health Center of Excellence (DHCoE) in order to promote development and innovation of digital technologies, which includes EHRs. The center serves patients, health providers, program developers, researchers, and industry and national and international bodies, as well as other centers within the FDA such as the Office of the National Coordinator for Health Information Technology (ONC) and CMS. The DHCoE promotes digital health empowerment through innovative regulatory approaches, partnership connections to accelerate digital health advancements, and knowledge sharing to increase understanding and best practice advancement.

Regulatory Billing Claims

There are regulations and guidelines that govern claims submission for health care services reimbursement. The EHR plays a critical role in billing for these claims as they serve as validation for services rendered. There are several regulatory billing claims that will be presented here that you must be knowledgeable of:

- CMS regulations: These regulations must be met in order for reimbursement to be awarded for services provided to patients. The EHR serves as a significant component in capturing and validating this information.
- **International Classification of Diseases (ICD) codes**: These text and number codes are the international standard used for systematic recording, reporting, analyzing, interpreting, and comparing mortality and morbidity data. It classifies diseases and medical conditions for billing and coding. Submission of these codes is required in order to receive reimbursement. The World Health Organization (WHO) designed the ICD system, and the U.S version was created by CMS and the National Center for Health Statistics (NCHS). ICD-11 is fully electronic, which means it can function in an EHR environment and link with terminologies like the Standardized Nomenclature of Medicine (SNOMED). It has extension codes that add relevant information to stem codes (Drösler et al., 2021) and allows for data clustering for added coding detail.

Reference: Drösler, S. E., Weber, S., & Chute, C. G. (2021). ICD-11 extension codes support detailed clinical abstraction and comprehensive classification. *BMC Medical Informatics and Decision Making*, *21*(278). https://doi.org/10.1186/s12911-021-01635-2

- **National Correct Coding Initiative (NCCI)**: Implemented by the CMS, it promotes national correct coding methodologies and serves to control improper coding to assure payment for services rendered that meet criteria. Correct coding assures correct payments for Medicare Part B and Medicaid health care provider claims. Procedure-to-Procedure (PTP) code pairs are reviewed or edited to prevent improper payment. A review of submitted claims may be denied following processing due to NCCI edits. CMS publicizes NCCI edits for public view at https://www.cms.gov/medicare-medicaid-coordination/national-correct-coding-initiative-ncci/ncci-medicaid/medicaid-ncci-edit-files.

- **Current Procedural Terminology (CPT) codes**: This is a uniform language maintained by the American Medical Association used to describe medical procedures and services received by patients. This allows for streamline reporting and increases accuracy and efficiency by health care providers. There are various types of codes under three categories. Category 1 is the largest and the most commonly used as it contains most of the procedure codes. Category 2 tracks performance management. Category 3 has codes for emergency and experimental procedures. This CPT language provides for accuracy and allows for faster billing processing as common standards and tracking codes are foundational for use.
- **Electronic Data Interchange (EDI) standards**: EDI in health care is a secure way to transmit information between institutions, insurers, and patients. All transmission entities follow specific data specifications, which allows conversion of information into nonhuman computer language, transmission, and then interpretation by the receiving computer. EDI in health care uses 10 types of HIPAA-compliant transactions:

    1. Health care claim transaction set = encounter information submission for claim.
    2. Retail pharmacy claim transaction = submission of retail pharmacy claims.
    3. Health care claim payment/advice transaction set = used by insurers to make payments or send advice to health care providers.
    4. Benefits enrollment and maintenance = used for member enrollment in a health care benefit plan by employers, government agencies, insurance agencies, or claims paying health care organizations.
    5. Payroll deducted and other group premium payment for insurance products = payments made for insurance products.
    6. Health care eligibility/benefit inquiry = health care institutions transmit queries regarding subscriber

(patient or dependent) eligibility for health care services to be rendered.

7. Health care eligibility/benefit response = answer to query regarding subscriber (patient or dependent) eligibility for health care services to be rendered.
8. Health care claim status request = request for update on status of a prior claim transaction sent for payment or action.
9. Health care claim status notification = report response on claim status previously provider submitted by health care payer and insurance company.
10. Health care service review information = used by hospitals to request payer authorization.

- Health Care Common Procedure Coding System (HCPCS): This is a set of standardized codes used for processing, billing, and reimbursement of health insurance claims. This common language promotes communication between health care providers, payers, and regulatory agencies. This system is maintained by CMS. HCPCS is divided into two levels: level I and level II. Level I is Current Procedural Terminology (CPT) codes that primarily describe clinical setting procedures and services. This system was developed and is maintained by the American Medical Association. Level II identifies products, services, supplies, durable medical equipment, and medications not included in CPT codes. This system is maintained by CMS.

The EHR promotes timely submission of essential, timely, and accurate information for reimbursement while facilitating compliance with federal requirements. Knowledge of these key components is critical to keep providers and organizations from receiving financial reductions in pay or penalties. Knowing expectations in order to facilitate development and updating of hardware and software to adhere to compliance requirements is just one of the many EHR specialist responsibilities.

Institute of Electrical and Electronics Engineers 1073 Standard for Medical Devices

The **Institute of Electrical and Electronics Engineers (IEEE)** family of standards and guidelines was developed to provide interoperable communication between medical devices that may be at a patient's bedside and the health care information computerized electronic system. The IEEE (n.d.) is an international technical professional organization dedicated to fostering innovation and advancing technology for the benefit of humanity. IEEE 1073 is specific to acute care and promotes comprehensive capturing of patient data from all connected devices to that patient. IEEE 1073 identifies that data captured from all patient devices will allow health care organizations to (a) design and improve treatment protocols; (b) allow remote access to real-time patient data from various locations by health care providers; (c) allow for real-time notification for medication intravenous infusion; (d) review real-time data analysis for medication effectiveness; (e) manage connected medical devices for location, manufacturer recall, and proper calibration; and (f) review real-time patient care changes to achieve costs reductions and improve health care (Kennelly, 1998).

References:

Institute of Electrical and Electronics Engineers. (n.d.). *Mission and vision*. https://www.ieee.org/about/vision-mission.html.

Kennelly, R. J. (1998). The IEEE 1073 Standard for Medical Device Communications [Paper presentation]. *IEEE Systems Readiness Technology Conference. Test Technology for the 21st Century*, Salt Lake City, UT. https://ieeexplore.ieee.org/document/713466

The 21st-Century Cures Act (Cures Act)

The **21st-Century Cures Act** was signed into law on December 13, 2016. An intent was to accelerate discovery, development, and delivery of cures in the 21st century. Another intent of this act was to promote interoperability of health information technology and prohibit information blocking to empower patients. It promoted the adoption of standardized application programming. This was designed to encourage interoperability across EHR vendors through the adoption of data exchange standards. The Information Blocking Provision of the Cures Act mandated that patients have free access to their electronic health information. Clear requirements for compliance by health care providers, institutions, health information exchanges, and vendors were cited with a mechanism for reporting violations through an information blocking portal on the ONC's website at https://inquiry.healthit.gov/support/plugins/servlet/desk/portal/6.

Chapter Summary

Understanding health care legislation and regulations is important to ensuring compliance, protecting patient privacy, and promoting quality delivery of care for the EHRS. HIPAA establishes standards for protecting individual health information and ensuring confidentiality, integrity, and availability. The HITECH Act promotes the adoption and meaningful use of EHRs for the improvement of quality, safe, and efficient health care. MACRA introduced payment reforms and quality reporting programs (e.g., MIPS, APMs). These incentivized value-based care to overall improve health care outcomes. It is important for the EHRS to understand how regulations and guidelines govern claims submission and reimbursement as well as the importance of accuracy and transparency of records. Meaningful Use is now known as the Medicare Promoting Interoperability Program and incentivizes eligible professionals and hospitals to effectively use certified EHR technology. The EHR is designed to improve care coordination, patient empowerment, and engagement in their care, and promote the exchange of health information. The Cures Act aims to accelerate medical innovation (research and technology) in order to enhance and improve quality of life. In combination, these legislative acts and regulatory frameworks serve to shape health care, drive progress, and improve patient outcomes.

6

FUNCTIONS AND TYPES OF EHR SYSTEMS

CHAPTER OBJECTIVES

Upon completion of this chapter, the reader will be able to do the following:

1. State components for the EHR provider portal and patient portal.
2. Define the two main types of EHR systems: (a) on-premises and (b) cloud-based.
3. Identify advantages and disadvantages for on-premises and cloud-based EHR systems.
4. Distinguish the types of EHR software and systems.
5. Identify critical security safeguards for the EHR system.

KEY CHAPTER TERMS

- Provider portal
- Patient portal
- On-premises
- Cloud-based
- Stand-alone systems
- Integrated systems
- Open-source software
- Specialty specific software
- Antivirus software
- Malware
- Security safeguards: administrative, physical, technical

Key Functions of the EHR System

EHRs have a variety of functions that promote health care provider patient management, which underlies improved patient care overall. These systems have two portal entries: one for the provider and one for the patient.

Provider Portal Entry Components

The **provider portal** is a web-based application that affords registered health care providers with the secure ability to input and retrieve patient information. Providers can also access information from other departments in order to provide interdisciplinary and specialized treatment. Portal components can allow the following and be expanded for specialty departments.

- Patient management information allows for input of patient data to manage problems and implement wellness activities. It provides a secure place for the patient demographics, medical history, laboratory results, interventional radiology results, medication history, and so on.
- Health care providers document clinical encounters, which include the chief complaint, diagnoses, treatment plans with medicinal prescriptions, and progress notes.
- Order management allows providers to manage patient orders in a fashion that reduces errors in duplicate orders by allowing medication reconciliation and identification of potential interactions.
- Laboratory and interventional tests are stored and forwarded to promote follow-up by the appropriate department. Orders and results for interventions used for decision-making are maintained, which can include tests, studies, and procedures. The program can filter out errors and duplicates in the system, which reduces overall costs and potential reimbursement issues.
- Decision support is achieved with the use of the EHR. The EHR has decision-making tools that allow for inquiries to potential diagnoses for ruling out specific diseases and identify a diagnosis from signs and symptoms. The search engine has protocols and research that promote provider-informed

patient care decisions. These are called Clinical Decision Support Systems (CDSS).

- Analytics and reporting information are obtained from the EHR through data retrieval. Obtaining data identifies trends in care. This allows for quality indicators to be validated or those identified needing further protocols for improvement. It identifies provider-specific information as well, which gives the governing organization information to improve outcomes for providers who may not be validating care as needed for reimbursement or the best outcomes possible.
- Communication that promotes interprofessional collaboration (between two or more members of different professions) and intra-professional collaboration (between two or more members within the same profession) is facilitated within the EHR provider portal. This portal promotes secure messaging between providers, which allows for the efficient and timely exchange of information. It allows for pictures and text messages to be exchanged via secure servers.
- Electronic prescribing portals that connect with pharmacies are possible. These allow for the care provider to communicate directly with local pharmacies. This function sends alerts and notifications regarding medication dosages, allergies, and possible drug interactions. This also promotes quick access to medications for patients.

Patient Portal Entry Components

Patients have direct access to their medical records by signing into a specific portal and entering a username and password after signing up. **Patient portals** allow care recipients the ability to access their health record. Information entered includes demographics, laboratory results, radiology results, diagnostic interventions, medication history, immunization record, allergies, diagnoses, visit notes, and so on. These sections of the record are locked and do not allow changes to be made by the patient. Communication sections are unlocked. These allow the patient to enter information that permits them to contact the physician for specific needs such as an interventional visit or medication renewal. This system also has the ability to send alerts or reminders to the patient regarding upcoming needs such as mammograms and bone density tests for wellness management.

Systems are generally maintained by independent care entities (e.g., hospitals, free-standing outpatient clinics, pharmacies, vision centers, etc.) that do not interact with one another. In order for care activities to be retrieved for entry into an individual patient record maintained by another organization, the patient must sign a request for information to be reported from one entity to the other (e.g., vision center records sent to the family practice clinic). Some systems have the ability to cross care provider specialties if they are maintained by a specific medical center or hospital with clinics (e.g., notes from dermatology, neurology, orthopedics, and the family practice physician are in one patient portal).

Types of EHR Systems

There are two main types of electronic records systems (a) on-premises (on prem) and (b) cloud based. There are also systems that combine the two, called hybrid systems. They might use on-premises systems for storing patient records and use the cloud-based system for patient portal access and e-prescribing services. The type of system will vary based on use such as (a) inpatient (hospital) versus outpatient (clinic) or (b) specialty specific (oncology, behavioral health) versus general practice (family practice). The ultimate decision usually comes down to needs and financial resources available for purchase as well as the capabilities of the EHR software system being investigated for use.

On-Premises EHR Systems

On-premises (on-prem) systems are located and run locally on the organization's own in-house servers and computers. All EHR data is stored on-site. These hardware and software components are serviced by the organizations' Information Technology (IT) department and team members. These systems have advantages and disadvantages (see Table 6.1).

TABLE 6.1 On-Premises Systems Do Have Their Advantages and Disadvantages

Advantages	Disadvantages
Anytime access (24/7)	Increased upfront costs (requires purchase of additional hardware, severs, computers)
Anywhere access (from patient room to across country) from various organizational locations	Increased IT department costs (must maintain expertise onsite for updates, system configuration and troubleshooting)
Offline operations possible (local access to system information when company makes changes to software)	Local data storage hardware subject to loss (environmental hazards such as fire, tornadoes, floods, etc. may result in loss of hardware where data is stored, which would result in loss of data)
Scheduled internet outages for updates (allows for outages to occur during off peak use times)	Limited scalability (software package sold as unit and organization must select and install select components)
Internal security (access to data believed to be better controlled)	Training may be left to IT personnel or other designated staff
	Required Business Associates Agreement (BAA) to maintain PHI security and overall HIPAA compliance may be nonrenewable

Cloud-Based EHR systems

Cloud-based systems are hosted remotely on a third-party vendor's servers and accessed via the internet. They have become more popular over the years, as capabilities of the internet have evolved. System overall costs are mainly determined by the number of organizational users and usage features required for servicing providers, patients, and data management. Most vendors will offer customization to allow an organization to select from an extensive list of available capabilities to promote efficient use, storage, and data retrieval. These systems have advantages and disadvantages (see Table 6.2).

TABLE 6.2 Cloud-Based Systems Do Have Their Advantages and Disadvantages

Advantages	Disadvantages
Anytime access (24/7)	Internet outages (update times not controlled by organization; outages due to loss of access for various reasons)
Anywhere access (from patient room to across country) from various organizational locations	Data security risks (information sent over the internet and kept at onsite servers subject to hackers and hijackers)
Reduced upfront cost (does not require on site hardware)	Increasing costs (cost of updates and software change implementation controlled by company)
Reduced onsite IT support required (smaller support team with smaller budget required for IT department)	
Scalable framework (software changes available at reduced implementation cost)	

Health Information Exchange

Health Information Exchange (HIE) is the electronic sharing of health care information between various providers and settings. These include hospitals, clinics, pharmacies, laboratories, providers, and so on. The HIE goal is to provide secure and interoperable exchange of patient health information to promote continuity and coordination of care delivery to ultimately reduce health care costs. It is not intended to replace provider–patient communication but enhance patient record completeness and promote joint review of care activities by patient and provider. There are three key forms of health information exchange, which include (a) directed exchange, in which care providers can send and receive secure information electronically; (b) query-based exchange, which gives providers the ability to locate or request specific information from other providers; and (c) consumer-mediated exchange, in which patients have the ability to aggregate and control the use of their health information. The HIE has advantages and disadvantages (see Table 6.3).

TABLE 6.3 **Health Information Exchange Advantages and Disadvantages**

Advantages	Disadvantages
Promotes improved health care provider coordination by giving health care providers access to information from other sources.	Privacy and security concerns as information open to potential unauthorized access and data breaches.
Reduces costs as it streamlines communication, which can prevent redundant tests and treatments required for patient intervention.	Various health care information systems and standards pose a challenge to interoperability.
Enhances patient safety through access to a comprehensive patient health record, which can promote identification of potential medication interactions, allergies, and potential adverse drug reactions.	Data quality and integrity between exchanged health information may lack accuracy and completeness, which can undermine usefulness and reliability of exchanged information.
Promotes continuity of care through accessibility to comprehensive patient health information.	Implementation and maintenance costs for infrastructure and systems may pose a limitation for smaller organizations and provider-based clinics.
Improves public health surveillance and reporting by giving public health agencies access to real-time data.	

Types of EHR Software and Systems

The EHR software market is vast worldwide. There are more than 500 companies offering some type of EHR software (Greene, 2021). Based on an examination of 5,400 hospitals, which were all acute care U.S.-based hospitals in 2018, the top software companies were

Epic and Oracle Cerner. The following was the market share division (Drees, 2019):

1. "Epic: 28 %
2. Cerner: 26 %
3. Meditech: 16 %
4. CPSI: 9 %
5. Allscripts: 6 %
6. Medhost: 4 %
7. athenahealth: 2 %
8. None/other: 9 %"

References:

Green, J. (2021). *Who are the largest EHR vendors?* EHR in Practice. https://www.ehrinpractice.com/largest-ehr-vendors.html

Drees, J. (2019, April 30). *KLAS: Epic, Cerner dominate EMR market share.* Becker's HealthIT. https://www.beckershospitalreview.com/ehrs/klas-epic-cerner-dominate-emr-market-share.html

There are different types of EHR systems and software: (a) **stand-alone systems**, (b) **integrated systems**, (c) **open-source software**, and (d) specialty **specific software**.

Stand-Alone EHR Systems

This type of system has specific components in one system. It is designed to stand alone or operate independently of other health care applications. It can be used to manage only specific aspects of a patient's health care information. For example, this system may be used to manage patient clinical health data such as the medical history, diagnoses, medications, allergies, and laboratory results. Other essential components, such as administrative and financial data, would be managed by a separate system.

The use of a stand-alone system means that administrative, clerical, health care providers and support must only master the use of one system. This can reduce time to implementation and full use capability by all individuals. These systems generally include keeping medical records as a main component. Other basic features include appointment scheduling and billing. These systems can run system-wide reports to validate meaningful use criteria and regulatory billing claims processing codes. Typically, the stand-alone system is used by smaller medical practices or specialty organizations. They may also be used to support other systems already purchased by an organization. This allows system expansion without the cost or time expenditure required for revising an entire software system.

One possible drawback to using this type of system is that it may not promote interprofessional collaboration in patient care. This is because it may not provide a complete view of a patient's health history. It compartmentalizes record components, so administrative or financial data may not be included in this system. This could result in gaps in health care or inefficiencies in care delivery. Ultimately the choice to select a stand-alone system will depend on the needs and goals of the organization or practice.

Integrated EHR Systems

This type of system has components in one centralized system. It is designed to integrate or combine health care applications. It has basic and advanced features and capabilities in one system. It results in a single comprehensive electronic record. This combined application typically includes clinical, administrative, and financial information related to a patient's health care stored in one database. It includes medical history, diagnoses, medications, allergies, lab results, imaging studies, and other relevant clinical data. The system can also include administrative information such as demographic data, insurance information, and billing and claims data. It, like all systems, can only be accessed by authorized organizational health care personnel.

Access to the complete patient record, including all components, is certainly an advantage of the integrated system. It allows real-time access and review by all care providers, which promotes interprofessional collaborative patient management. This can improve quality and safety by ensuring that providers have access to all relevant information needed to make an informed decision about diagnoses, treatments, and ongoing care.

Overall, an integrated EHR system can improve the quality and efficiency of health care delivery as it provides a comprehensive view of the patient. This system saves time and decreases errors as it reduces manual input of data and hard copy retrieval of information from other system components needed for decision-making. This total view promotes efficient and cost-effective health care delivery through a streamlined administrative and billing process.

Open-Source EHR Software

Open-source EHR software is software that is free to download and use. This software is typically made available to the public without cost, or restrictions and the source code can be retrieved and modified by users to customize it to their organizational needs.

This EHR software is usually developed by a community of developers. They collaborate on the software project, contributing code and documentation, which improves the software over time. This collaborative approach brings together developers with varying levels of expertise, which can result in a more robust and customizable software product. The combined knowledge allows for identification of bugs with expert fixes, and even additions of new features, more quickly and efficiently.

Affordability is one advantage of open-source EHR software. It is cheaper than proprietary software as there are no licensing fees or other costs associated with use. Users have more control over the software because the source code is available to anyone. Being open source allows organizations the freedom to make program modifications to meet their specific needs.

Another benefit is that it is more flexible and customizable than proprietary software. Users can control customizability through source code modification. This requires organizations to have an IT department with individuals trained in software architecture. These IT specialists can alter codes to meet specific workflows and organization or clinic requirements. They can also add new features and integrate current systems into the open-source software package.

Overall, open-source EHR software can be cost-effective and customizable. This solution can facilitate implementation for small offices and organizations with limited resources. However, it may require the organization to hire individuals with more technical expertise and resources not necessarily required for proprietary software because those who use this open-source software must maintain and update the software themselves.

Specialty-Specific EHR Software

Specialty EHR software is software that is designed for a specific purpose. These are generally used by medical specialties such as pediatrics, oncology, cardiology, neurology, optometry, dentistry, behavioral health, or dermatology. This software typically uses specialized features and templates tailored to the needs of the specific medical specialty. These needs are identified by organizational goals and intent and the health care needs of users. Factors that play into specialty-specific EHR software selection include organizational size, budget constraints, and the specific medical specialty.

Specialty software can be tailored to address the needs of specialties and subspecialties. For example, these software programs can address cardiology as a major specialty and pediatrics as a subspecialty. This way, features and templates have specific order sets, documentation templates, and clinician decision tools to not only address cardiology but management of pediatric patients with cardiac conditions. This allows for streamlined workflows with error detection specific to pediatric cardiac medications, procedures, and so on. This promotes more effective and efficient care delivery.

Specialty-specific software can have features that allow for integration into other software systems within the organization. These can include medical imaging systems, laboratory information systems, or billing and coding software. This can help health care providers to manage unique clinical and administrative specialty requirements more easily and efficiently. The bottom line is that care quality is improved, errors are reduced, and efficiency is promoted and achieved.

One possible drawback to specialty-specific EHR software is that it may not be as customizable as a more general system. Flexibility is limited as the provider must work within the constraints of the software with limited ability to easily modify it. If the provider works in multiple specialties, it will be necessary for them to learn and manage multiple EHR systems based on the specialty they are working in at any given time. This can certainly be challenging.

Antivirus Software

Antivirus software is important to protect not only PHI components but also the system itself. Antivirus software protects by detecting, preventing, and removing malicious software (**malware**) from a computer and other critical devices that house the EHR and other PHI. Malware can include viruses, trojans, adware, spyware, and other programs that can harm or steal information (e.g., hijacking information for ransom). Antivirus software can scan and remove or prevent malware from being installed. There are many antivirus options that may come as stand-alone products or as part of a security suite. Options are often determined by facility administration and departmental leaders, which may include recommendations from the Chief Security Officer, if that role exists within the organization.

Security Safeguards

Research has identified three main **security safeguards** which are **administrative**, **physical**, and **technical**, to secure personal health information (PHI; Kruse et al., 2017) (see Table 6.4). These directly relate to the HIPAA Security Rule, which requires safeguards to ensure confidentiality, integrity, and security for PHI. Administrative safeguards are focused on compliance with policies and procedures directly related to the EHR, which include selection, development, implementation, and maintenance of PHI security measures. Physical safeguards are focused on protection of physical access through specific hardware and software controls for workstations and other access devices. Technical safeguards are focused on data and information systems where the PHI resides. All safeguards have specific terms associated with them (see Table 6.5). Various strategies can be implemented to address each of these security safeguards.

TABLE 6.4 Security Safeguards

Administrative	Physical	Technical
• Risk analysis/ assessment [1,2]	• Access controls [1,2]	• Encryption [1,2]
• Security policy [2]	• Workstation security [1,2]	• Audit [1,2] and monitor [2]
• Disaster recovery plan [1]	• Data backup management [2]	• Firewall [1]
• Training [2]		• Virus protection [1]

References:

[1] Kruse, C. S., Smith, B., Vanderlinden, H., & Nealand, A. (2017). Security techniques for the electronic health records. *Journal of Medical Systems, 41*(8), 127. https://doi.org/10.1007/s10916-017-0778-4

[2] Medical Information Technology Group. (2022, May 10). *Best electronic health record (EHR) security measures.* Medical ITG. https://medicalitg.com/electronic-health-record-security-measures/

TABLE 6.5 Security Safeguard Terms Defined

Administrative

Term	Definition
Risk analysis/ assessment	Identifying and evaluating for potential threats (e.g., cyberattack) that may negatively affect an organization and its operations
Security policy	A document that outlines a planned procedure and/or administrative action of what to do for an organization in the event of a danger or threat to protect itself
Disaster recovery plan	A document that identifies steps to be taken in the event of a potential disaster that would affect the organization
Training	The action of teaching with the intent to increase knowledge and/or skills related to a particular job

Physical

Term	Definition
Access controls	Data security processes designed to restrict the ability of a person to access, manage, or edit specific data based on their level of authority or job description
Workstation security	Measures taken to maintain the safety of information on equipment designed to meet requirements for employees to perform specialized tasks related to designated jobs. Designed to address information on workstations that may be mobile or stationary
Data backup management	A continuous process of replication where data is copied on a regular basis to other systems within or outside of an organization to ensure a current, reliable, and accessible stored copy of accurate data and information exists. May use a third party–managed service provider (MSP) that remotely performs this process

Technical

Term	Definition
Encryption	Computerized information security protection process that scrambles information from plain text into an unreadable format (cyphertext) so that only an authorized individual with the key can unscramble (decryption) and read it
Audit	An official inspection or examination of an organization's information technology infrastructure and applications. This can be expanded to include data use and management, policies and procedures, and operational processes
Monitor	To observe (keep under systematic review) and check for quality or compliance
Firewall	Software that examines traffic into and out of a computer network system to determine safety. If firewall standards are met, traffic will be allowed to pass through to the user
Virus protection	Antivirus software that protects by detecting, preventing, and removing malicious software (malware) from a computer and other critical devices

Chapter Summary

It is imperative that the EHRS understand numerous EHR provider components. The provider portal entry allows authorized health care professionals to access and manage patient health record components. The patient portal enables patients to securely assess their health information, communicate with their provider, and schedule appointments as a participant in their own care. EHR systems can be categorized into two main types: on premises (on-prem) and cloud based. On premises are housed and managed within the organization's infrastructure. This affords greater system control but can require a significant upfront investment and continued maintenance. Cloud-based systems are hosted and maintained by a third-party vendor on remote servers. This affords scalability, flexibility, and accessibility from any location with an internet access but can have data security concerns and depends on external service provider quality. Diverse types of EHR software and systems are available, and each is tailored to meet specific organizational needs and preferences. Critical security safeguards include encryption, access controls and user authentication, audit trails for activity and unauthorized use detection, software patches and updates to address potential security vulnerabilities, and backup systems for disaster data recovery. It is important for the EHRS to understand these EHR components, types, advantages, disadvantages, and security safeguards in order to promote making informed decisions to select, implement, and maintain solutions that provide the efficient and effective delivery of care within their specific organization.

7

EHR COMPONENTS

CHAPTER OBJECTIVES

Upon completion of this chapter, the reader will be able to do the following:

1. Identify various EHR components.
2. Define various EHR components.
3. Analyze Protected Health Information (PHI) data.
4. Interpret various types of EHR documentation components.

KEY CHAPTER TERMS

- Demographic information
- Clinical record
- Medication Administration Record (MAR)
- Diagnoses
- Laboratory reports
- Physician Orders for Scope of Treatment (POST)
- Protected Health Information (PHI)
- Subjective, Objective, Assessment, Plan (SOAP)
- Imaging
- Operative reports
- Discharge summary
- History and physicals

EHR Components

The EHR is a digital system that organizes a patient's medical information into a centralized location. It includes several key components (see Table 7.1).

TABLE 7.1 EHR Components and Explanations

EHR Component	Explanation
Demographic information	This section includes personal details such as patient name, contact information, gender, date of birth, and emergency contacts (family or friends). Patient insurance information (primary insurance, secondary insurance, policy numbers, group numbers) is also in this section.
Clinical record	This record includes the medical history (current and past illnesses, medical conditions, surgical procedures, and chronic conditions). This area also includes any clinical notes from a care provider (e.g., SOAP notes, physician notes, clinical notes).
Medication Administration Record (MAR)	This record includes all medications the patient is currently prescribed. This comprehensive list incorporates all medications ordered for patient treatment inclusive of medication names, dosages prescribed for administration, times for medication administration, and routes of administration (oral, intramuscular, intravenous, topical, per nasogastric tube, etc.). Documentation of medication administration is also validated in this record by the provider. Most MARs directly interact with the EHR through a barcode system and as medications are administered, they are automatically electronically validated in the patient record.

(Continued)

TABLE 7.1 (*Continued*)

EHR Component	Explanation
Diagnoses	This section includes the determination and identification of the patient's specific disease or condition based on a preexisting set of categories. The diagnoses and diagnostic codes are identified often using the International Classification of Diseases (ICD) codes. Clinical terms coded with ICD are the basis for health recordkeeping and allow for data retrieval and statistical analyses on societal diseases. A diagnosis is required to determine a treatment plan and tracking of a patient's medical history. It is also required for insurance claims and payment.
Laboratory reports	This section contains diagnostic test results. These are results from blood tests, urinalyses, imaging studies, diagnostic tests, and pathology reports. These are used to determine diagnoses and validate treatment options.
Orders	This section is where health care providers write instructions (orders) to be followed to promote care delivery and facilitate health and wellness. These are orders for interventions that can include treatments, diagnostic tests, medications, and specialist referrals. These orders can be electronically transmitted directly to the appropriate department. • POST form: This stands for **Physician Orders for Scope of Treatment** form. This is an order set based on the patient's condition and advanced directives. It actually puts the patient's advanced directives into action by setting them up as a physician's medical order. This allows for continuity of actions related to a patient's wishes and ensures that there is transfer of this information across care settings.

EHR Component	Explanation
Billing information	This section is where financial information is maintained. This includes details for insurance company reimbursement (procedure codes and diagnostic codes). Accurate information and billing codes must be submitted for reimbursement to prevent refusal of payment for care delivery (refusal due to paperwork technicality). Refusal may also occur due to lack of coverage for a specific intervention, liability dispute, or preexisting medical condition or injury.

Protected Health Information

What is **protected health information (PHI)**? PHI is essentially any information collected or generated by a health care provider that represents past, present, or future mental or physical patient or client conditions. This is information that is identifiable in an individual health record maintained or transmitted in any medium (oral, written, or electronic format). The PHI can be abbreviated as ePHI when information is in electronic format. It can be maintained by an entity or an associate of the entity. The Health Insurance Portability and Accountability Act (HIPAA) privacy rule has a very clear definition for PHI. The privacy rule is located at 45 CFR Part 160 and Subparts A and E of Part 164. It defines PHI as any information that can be used to identify an individual's health status, treatment given for conditions (physical or psychological), or payment used for health care services. PHI includes demographic information (name, address, age, race, gender, etc.), medical history (diagnoses, treatments, etc.), test results (blood, radiological, etc.), insurance information, and other data that can be used to identify specific patients.

PHI can be disclosed if it is de-identified. This means that it must be stripped of all identifying information that would allow it to be linked to a specific patient. If identifiers are removed, the information is considered de-identified PHI. HIPAA does not apply to this de-identified PHI, and the information can be disclosed without violating HIPAA rules. This may be done if the data is used as grouped data for statistical analyses or quality improvement, for example.

There are situations when PHI can be released without patient consent. These include providers participating in treatment and care, businesses that provide services to participating providers, or billing institutions. PHI can also be released related to public health and safety concerns and if related to legal action before a court (e.g., court litigation), for arbitration, or to an administrative agency by subpoena or in response to a legal discovery request (e.g., coroner's investigation).

PHI policies are important for the protection of all patient information. All employees must be aware of the policies and procedures required to not only safeguard patients but the organization, as violations can result in stiff fines and even employee termination.

Types of Health Care Documentation

Health care documentation includes **Subjective, Objective, Assessment, Plan (SOAP)** progress notes; laboratory reports; imaging records; operative reports; orders directed for care by the provider; discharge summaries from inpatient or outpatient care; and the patient history and physical. All have their specific place in the EHR. These are critical to individual and interdisciplinary health care provider patient management.

- *Subjective, Objective, Assessment, Plan (SOAP) progress notes* are a structured method of recording patient information. It allows for a systematic record of patient information and is used among many providers, including physicians, nurses, therapists, and other care clinicians. It incorporates several data components. This patient data organizational component allows for a clear and concise manner of patient data retrieval and validation.
    - Subjective: This type of documentation includes validation of patient's symptoms identified verbally, personal feelings related to their situation, and any concerns voiced or expressed in any manner to the care provider. In real terms this is information the patient verbally communicates to the health care provider.
    - Objective: This type of documentation includes data that is observed, measurable, and factual. This includes physiological measurements such as vital signs (temperature, heart rate, respiratory rate, and blood

pressure). Physical examination findings (findings from the physical review of body systems) and observable signs (e.g., effort of breathing) may be recorded here. Diagnostic results relative to the patient's reason for seeking care may also be placed in this area.

- Assessment: This type of documentation includes the health care provider's synthesis of the data in prior areas (subjective and objective). This synthesis results in the decision of a diagnosis and/or differential diagnosis. If the patient is returning for a follow-up care visit, this area can be used to validate a response to treatment or progress toward a designated health care goal. Clinical reasoning and medical expertise are used as the foundation for decisions in this documentation area.
- Plan: This type of documentation includes the plan of care designed by the health care provider to promote wellness and recovery derived from the synthesis of all pertinent information and information under assessment. This detailed plan includes a treatment plan, interventions, medications, additional diagnostic tests, referrals to specialized care providers, and any follow-up requirements to be implemented in order to promote health, wellness, or recovery. Ideally this plan includes collaboration with the patient for implementation.

- *Laboratory reports* are results from tests used to examine cells or measure chemicals or other substances in body fluids. The EHR maintains reports sequentially to allow comparisons and facilitate identification of normal or abnormal trends. These are used to determine diagnoses and validate treatment options as well as outcomes of interventions for diseases.
- ***Imaging*** is a medical procedure that uses various techniques to create detailed pictures of various internal body parts for the purpose of identifying abnormalities, facilitating a diagnosis, and identifying and validating procedural interventions. All are noninvasive, which means that they can produce internal body images (usually digital) from outside the body with no requirements to enter a body cavity. Digital Imaging and Communications in Medicine (DICOM) is the international standard for medical images

and related information data and quality exchange. This standard identifies formats for medical images to ensure quality for clinical use. The Picture Archiving and Communication System (PACS) is a computerized method for replacing conventional radiological films. In this system radiological images are acquired, stored, transmitted, and digitally displayed. PACS allows the generation of a filmless clinical environment.

- The five most common types of imaging tests are as follows:
  - X-rays use electromagnetic radiation to generate images of bones and various tissue based on density. More dense structures appear lighter (bones appear very light, the liver would appear light) and less dense structures appear darker (lungs are air filled and appear very dark).
  - Computed tomography (CT) scans use multiple X-ray images and combine them with the aid of a computer to generate detailed images of internal body structures. These images are taken from different angles and use computer processing to generate cross-sectional images called slices, that appear as pictures. This scan can also be called a CAT scan, which stands for computed axial tomography.
  - Nuclear medicine scans use a small amount of radiation (radioactive tracers) to generate images of bones, tissues, and body organs. Examples of the most common scans include Single-Photon Emission Computed Tomography (SPECT) and Positive Emission Tomography (PET). They can be used to identify tumors and other abnormalities. Even though they may identify an abnormality, other more focused tests are required for a more definitive diagnosis of cancer (e.g., biopsy where a small part of the tissue is removed and examined for abnormal cells).
  - Ultrasound uses sound waves with frequencies higher than the upper limits audible to the human ear to generate a two-dimensional image for examining internal body structures and detecting abnormalities. It is especially used in maternity care to view fetal development.
  - Medical Resonance Imaging (MRI) scans use strong magnetic fields, magnetic field gradients, and computer-generated radio waves to generate images of internal

body components. This large tube-shaped machine can form pictures of not just the anatomy but the physiological processes of the body. It can produce cross-sectional images like slices in a loaf of bread. It can also generate three-dimensional images that can be viewed from various angles.

- *Operative reports* are summaries of surgical procedures. The operative report includes the preoperative diagnosis, postoperative diagnosis, findings of the surgical procedure, the procedure used for the specific operation, identification of any problems encountered during the procedure and the postoperative condition of the patient prior to recovery. These summaries support the need for the surgical intervention procedure as well as the results.
- *Orders* are where health care providers write instructions (orders) to be followed to promote care delivery and facilitate health and wellness. These include orders for interventions that can include treatments, diagnostic tests, medications, and specialist referrals. These orders can be electronically transmitted directly to the appropriate department.
- *Discharge summaries* are clinical reports generated at the conclusion of a hospital stay. This clinical synopsis serves as the primary method of communication for transition to aftercare providers for patient continuity of care and promotion of a successful treatment regimen. These final diagnostic statements outline details of the patient's hospital stay and are required to be completed within 30 days (organizations may require earlier posting). These documents are regulated by the Joint Commission (formally called Joint Commission on Accreditation of Healthcare Organizations [JCAHO]), which is responsible for accreditation of health care organizations. The Joint Commission mandates this synopsis include: (a) the reason for hospitalization, (b) significant findings, (c) procedures/treatments provided, (d) condition at discharge, (e) instructions to patient and family (if applicable), and (f) electronic attending physician's signature. The discharge summary is closely aligned with coding and billing.
- *History and Physicals* (H&Ps) are complete assessments of a patient and the problem they present with for care. The H&P is written by a physician or qualified licensed practitioner

who has this ability within their scope of practice by law and regulation. Some population groups have specific history and physical requirements based on the Joint Commission, which include behavioral health homes, opioid treatment programs, children and youth, individuals with intellectual/development disabilities, eating disorders, and addictions treatment. Other required content to be included in the H&P may be determined by the organization based on setting, service, and population served. The Joint Commission requires that the H&P be completed no more than 30 days prior to a patient's admission and within 24 hours after an admission but before a surgical treatment.

Chapter Summary

EHR components vary by system and purpose for specific organizations. These include modules for capturing, storing, and accessing patient health care data such as demographics, medical history, allergies, medications, laboratory results, and diagnostic radiological images. Each facilitates clinical documentation, care coordination, and decision-making by members of the interprofessional health care team. Any information transmitted and maintained is subject to privacy and security regulations under HIPAA. PHI must be handled appropriately and in accordance with HIPAA requirements. Various types of EHR documentation components include but are not limited to SOAP progress notes, laboratory reports, imaging studies, operative reports, and orders. These serve to provide a comprehensive record of patient encounters, treatments, and outcomes. They promote continuity of care and validate reimbursements for services. By understanding and effectively using EHR components the EHRS can enhance organizational outcomes and facilitate compliance with regulatory requirements.

8

MEDICAL DATABASES AND MANAGEMENT SYSTEMS

CHAPTER OBJECTIVES

Upon completion of this chapter, the reader will be able to do the following:

1. Discriminate between primary and secondary databases for health care organizations.
2. Define one of the more common database management systems in health care.
3. Differentiate database systems based on requirements and structure.

KEY CHAPTER TERMS

- Primary database
- Secondary database
- Document database
- Hierarchical Database Management System (DBMS)
- Network DBMSs
- Relational Database Management System (RDBMS)
- Object-oriented Database (OOD)
- Proprietary systems for database housing

Medical Databases

Databases play a critical role in health care as they organize and allow for dissemination of information in a format that is understandable. The following is general information for databases, but there can be any number of databases from an organization: administrative (employee database), specific to a designated unit (critical care database), or specific to a care delivery component (cardiovascular congestive heart failure database). This will depend on the organization and its ability to not only generate but maintain such databases.

Primary and Secondary Databases

Primary and secondary databases are unique and different in their intent and purpose. The primary can be purposed for an individual organization but a secondary can be derived from various health care organizations. While they are both databases, it is imperative that the EHRS know the difference.

- The **primary database** is built by the health care organization. It can also be a primary repository held by an entity. These databases contain information collected firsthand by the organization and maintained as part of their data used for analyses and quality improvement initiatives. Some primary database examples include the following:
    - EHR systems store primary comprehensive electronic health records for patients such as demographic information, medical history, medications, imaging reports, surgical interventions, and so on.
    - Clinical Trial Databases are primary repositories of clinical data collected for research studies such as subjects, interventions, outcomes, adverse events, and so on.
    - Registries collect and maintain standardized data on specific diseases, conditions, treatments, or populations (e.g., cancer registries, implant registries, diabetes registries, etc.).
    - Laboratory information systems manage and report patient results (e.g., test orders, specimens, results, etc.).

- The **secondary database** is made up of various health care organizations that provide patient clinical information. These include hospitals, clinics, physician groups, and insurance companies. This data is retrieved from primary sources, analyzed, and can be used for comparison of trends among various organizations and for identification of needed community initiatives. Some secondary database examples include the following:
  - Health insurance claims databases serve to allow analysis and utilization management of services and include information on health care services provided to patients and reimbursed by insurance companies. This secondary data can include medical claims, billing codes, procedures, diagnoses, and amounts reimbursed for care interventions.
  - National health surveys collect data on health-related behaviors, risk factors, and outcomes from population samples for epidemiological studies and health policy development. A few examples include the National Health and Nutrition Examination Survey (NHANES), the Behavioral Risk Factor Surveillance System (BRFSS), and the National Health Interview Survey (NHIS).
  - Disease registries aggregate disease and condition data from various sources to track prevalence, incidence, and outcomes. A few examples include state-based cancer registries, cardiovascular disease registries, and infectious disease surveillance systems.

Document Databases

These databases are maintained to house important information such as legal, medical, employee, or other types of records that must be kept by an organization. These databases are structured to allow for easy access and retrieval of documents in various formats (Portable Document Format [PDF], video, PowerPoints, etc.). They also allow for security and safety against loss and access by individuals who should not be able to retrieve this information. **Document databases** allow employees with access to obtain key information for reports and other required quality improvement initiatives.

Database Management Systems

Database models can differ based on specific needs and characteristics of a health care organization. The following are some of the common database models used in the health care industry.

Hierarchical Database Management System

A **hierarchical database management system (DBMS)** resembles a tree in that the data is organized in a tree-like structure or parent–child relationship node hierarchy (see Figure 8.1). It will have a single root node, which is the parent (the topmost node) and which branches out into several child nodes (one to many relationships). Data is stored in fields, and each field contains only one value. An advantage to this structure is that it is easy to rapidly access and update. A disadvantage is that relationships between children are not allowed.

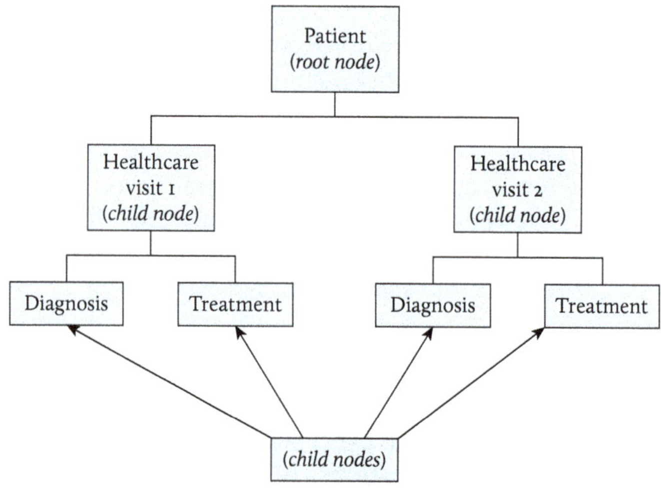

FIGURE 8.1 Hierarchical DBMS.

Network DBMS

Network DBMSs create a relationship between entities using a network structure. The Network DBMS is hierarchical, but instead of just one parent this type of database uses a network node system that can have multiple entity relationships. This makes the system look more like a cobweb instead of a tree (see Figure 8.2). In this database parents are called occupiers, and children are called members. In this system the child (called a member) can have more than one parent (called an occupier). This is a one-to-many system. Advantages to this structure are that it is relatively simple to design, it is a one-to-many design structure, there is easy data access (easier than the hierarchical one), and it can better isolate programs. Disadvantages are the complexity of the system as it is based on pointers to various components, and it is not easy to delete, insert, or update records due to the number of pointer adjustments that may be required due to the one-to-many structure.

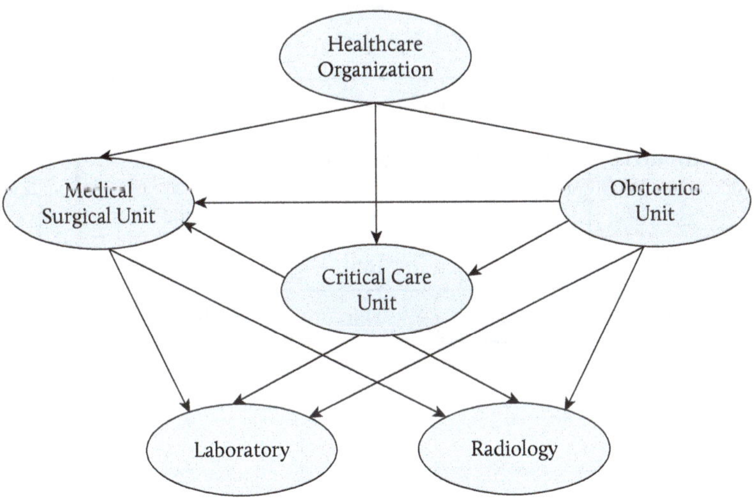

FIGURE 8.2 Network DBMS.

Relational Database Management System

A **relational database management system (RDBMS)** has data organized in rows and columns (e.g., two-dimensional table) (see Table 8.1). The relationship is maintained through common field storage. It can be used to track various forms of treatments, outcomes, and clinical indicators. It is called relational because the data items within them have predetermined relationships with one another. This system can be linked to various other EHR components that would automatically insert information when entered in other systems into the RDBMS (e.g., the relational database in the coronary care intensive care unit [CCICU] can be linked to the admission database, so information is entered in the CCICU database when admission information is entered).

- Rows in the table records are called tuples or records. These represent individual instances in the data.
- Columns in the table are called attributes. They represent data categories.
- Primary keys are the unique identifiers (key) for each row. Tables can be linked using these keys.

TABLE 8.1 Relational Database

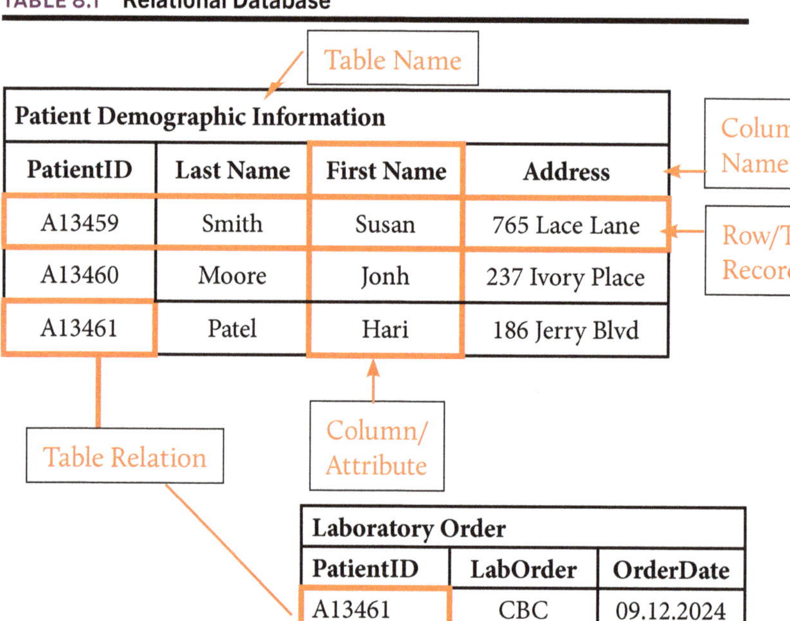

Patient Demographic Information			
PatientID	**Last Name**	**First Name**	**Address**
A13459	Smith	Susan	765 Lace Lane
A13460	Moore	Jonh	237 Ivory Place
A13461	Patel	Hari	186 Jerry Blvd

Laboratory Order		
PatientID	**LabOrder**	**OrderDate**
A13461	CBC	09.12.2024

Many relational databases use Structured Query Language (SQL). This domain specific language is used in design and programming. This language specifically allows interactions with a database, specifically the RDBMS. Some examples of relational databases are the Oracle Database which is a multi-model database management system by Oracle Corporation; MySQL an open-source (free) relational database that runs on almost all platforms (e.g., Linux, UNIX, Windows); and Microsoft SQL Server, which supports business and analytic applications. Advantages include its popularity; the ability to allow revisions of table information that is easy to understand;

and due to the fact that it supports data independence and structure independence design, maintenance and administration of the model is easier than the two prior database models. A disadvantage includes the difficulty in mapping objects in this database. This type is better suited for small databases, and the integrity of the data can be difficult to ensure due to the relational component.

Object-Oriented Database

An **object-oriented database (OOD)** can work with complex data objects. These are objects that may be used in object-oriented programming. Unlike other databases, the OOD can handle different types of data, which can include graphics (pictures) and video in addition to numbers and text, which is an advantage. It can encapsulate or group data into a single object. In the OOD objects are assigned a class. This class verifies both hierarchy (super-class or subclass) and functionality. Classes are groups of objects with the same properties and behaviors. Objects also have properties or attributes and behaviors, which are called methods, actions, or functions. Behaviors can modify or operate properties. This can make the OOD more complex in comparison to other types of database management systems—a disadvantage (see Figure 8.3).

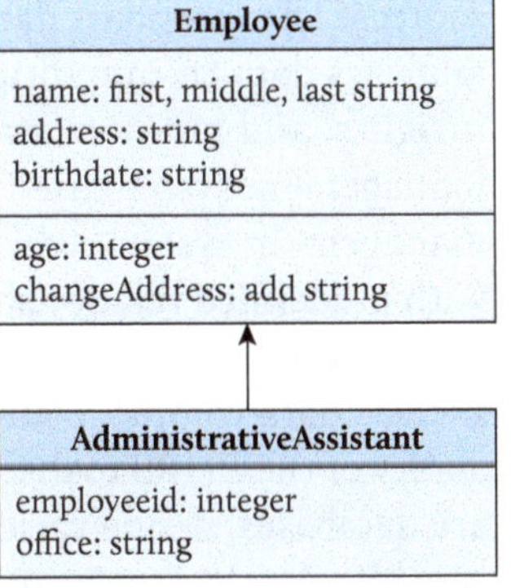

FIGURE 8.3 Object-oriented database.

Proprietary Systems for Database Housing

Proprietary systems for database housing are those that are privately owned by organizations but commercially licensed. These systems are specifically designed for a designated health care organization. Although there are definite advantages to this type of system (customizable for specific needs, scalable to handle large quantities of data, seamless integration into other organization systems, vendor support), they come with disadvantages (cost due to licensing fees and maintenance expenses; updates and support locked in by the vendor, which can make switching expensive and time-consuming; limited company transparency regarding algorithms and system architecture).

Chapter Summary

Understanding database distinctions is important for the EHRS to effectively manage and utilize their data assets. The primary database contains original, real-time data collected directly from sources. The secondary database, on the other hand, aggregates and analyzes data from multiple primary sources to generate trends, insights, and promote statistical analyses. A common database management system used in health care is the relational database management system, which organizes data into structured tables with predefined relationships between entities. Database systems can be differentiated based on their requirements and structure such as data volume, complexity, security, and performance. The ability of the EHRS to discriminate between primary and secondary databases, define various database management systems, and consider database requirements and structure will allow them to facilitate effective decisions about organizational data management strategies, technology investments, and resource allocations.

9

LATEST EHR TRENDS

CHAPTER OBJECTIVES

Upon completion of this chapter, the reader will be able to do the following:

1. Define interoperability as it relates to the EHR.
2. Summarize the effect of Artificial Intelligence on the EHR.
3. Distinguish patient-generated health care data.
4. Describe telehealth technologies.
5. Recognize blockchain technology.

KEY CHAPTER TERMS

- Interoperability
- Artificial Intelligence
- Blockchain technology
- Patient-generated health data
- Telehealth
- Telemedicine
- Fast Health care Interoperability Resources (FHIR)

Latest EHR Industry Trends

The EHR industry is constantly evolving. This evolution results in new trends and applications that promote increased security, usability, and improved functionality. They are being explored and used to improve patient care and outcomes.

Interoperability

Interoperability is the ability for different EHR systems to exchange patient information. In May 2020, CMS published the Interoperability and Patient Access final rule (CMS-9115-F), which emphasized the need to improve the exchange of health care information in order to achieve appropriate and complete health records for patients, health care providers, as well as organizations. It also facilitated the provision of patient-centered care through the improvement of prior authorization processes.

The Office of the National Coordinator for Health Information Technology (ONC) is the principal federal entity charged with coordination of nationwide efforts to implement and use the most advanced health information technology specifically for the exchange of health information. The ONC was established in 2004 by executive order from President George W. Bush. Congress later legislatively mandated the ONC in the Health Information Technology for Economic and Clinical Health Act (HITECH Act) of 2009 under President Obama's administration.

The ONC published new U.S. Core Data for Interoperability (USCDI) standards in January 2024. The USCDI (2024) "is a standardized set of data elements for nationwide, interoperable health information exchange" (para. 1). This draft version 5 identifies several new data classes and elements. The final version is targeted for release in July 2024.

Reference: U.S. Core Data for Interoperability. (2024, January). *United States core data for interoperability*. https://www.healthit.gov/isa/sites/isa/files/2024-01/Draft-USCDI-Version-5-January-2024-Final.pdf

Artificial Intelligence

In the future, **artificial intelligence** (AI) and the patient electronic health record are likely to be integrated into collaborative systems. AI is already being used in medical education and in operating suites during surgical procedures. One potential application is the use of AI to develop treatment care algorithms and identify potential diagnoses. AI will have the potential, through electronic health record integration, to analyze large amounts of data to develop potential diagnoses from a list of abstract symptoms that the patient may exhibit. This can assist health care providers in making more accurate and timely diagnoses. It may allow treatment plans to be individualized based on unique patient characteristics.

AI can also be used in the electronic health record to retrieve data from written text language by developing algorithms for extraction of themes and important data. Text information is unstructured and may be written in other languages. AI will have the potential to translate and extract information to allow the provider to develop unique treatment plans for each patient more easily.

"In addition to AI, other emerging technologies such as blockchain and the Internet of Things (IoT) may also play a role in the future of EHRs. For example, blockchain technology could be used to securely and efficiently share patient data between different healthcare providers, while IoT devices such as wearables or implantable sensors could provide real-time data on patient health that could be integrated into EHRs" (OpenAI, 2023).

Reference: OpenAI. (2023). *ChatGPT* (Mar 14 version) [Large language model]. https://chat.openai.com/chat

AI and electronic health record integration will certainly increase in the future. This improved sophistication will lead to improved patient outcomes and more efficient and effective collaborative health care delivery. Even though AI has proven and will continue to prove beneficial to patient care, it has its pitfalls and will pose challenges as all technology has in the past and will do in the future. Concerns will continue to exist about data security, privacy, and ownership. Oversight will continue to evolve as the need for policies, procedures, and regulations persists.

Blockchain Technology

Blockchain technology is being explored as a way to improve and increase the security of systems. It is a peer-to-peer (P2P) decentralized system compared to the current centralized systems where data is stored. This distributed and public ledger records transactions and makes records of any digital information that is transparent and unchangeable. It does not involve any third-party intermediary for security. It makes and generates a retroactively unchangeable record. The only way changes can be made is to initiate a change in all subsequent blocks with network consensus. Blockchain is thought to offer greater security compared to networks that are the traditional client-server based.

Patient-Generated Health Data

Patient-generated health data is being produced through wearable devices and on carried devices with computer applications such as smartphones. These devices promote patient engagement in their own health and health record data generation. They improve patient self-care activities, which ultimately can lead to healthier outcomes. These devices help patients take a more active role in their own health and wellness as they provide real-time progress feedback. The ability to track healthy lifestyle activities over time can improve an individual's desire to continue activities that promote successful outcomes.

Patient-generated health care data devices can track and record data related to heart rate, sleep patterns, and exercise frequency and intensity. These technologies continue to improve and evolve as computer capabilities expand. As these improvements become more widespread it is possible that this data generated through patient wearable and carried devices will integrate with the patients EHR. This data may subsequently be used to generate a more complete history of daily patterns and activities that can help the provider diagnose problems and make more informed treatment decisions. Integration of this data into the patient EHR can promote more patient and provider awareness of activities that affect health and overall well-being.

Despite the many advantages to these devices there are challenges. One is that the person wearing the device may not be the patient, resulting in the input of inaccurate data into the patient record when there is a direct link from the patient device to their EHR. Another is that the device, as well as the EHR, may be subject to data breaches and security risks as there is an open link between the two.

Just as technology has evolved over the past several years, patient-wearable devices and applications will continue to evolve. It will be important for the health care provider, and all involved with EHR data, to remain aware of changes and stay up-to-date on phases of these developments. Patients, providers, administrators, technology companies, and policymakers will need to work together to ensure that all can take full advantage of these technological benefits while minimizing risks.

Telehealth

Telehealth is the use of electronic information and telecommunication technologies to support the delivery of health-related services and information over long distances in a virtual format that supports patient care, administrative activities, and access to health care services. Virtual visits incorporate live communications with one's actual care provider. Telehealth allows for health care to be administered via telecommunication components (video conferencing and secure messaging) between patient and professional for the purpose of care delivery and health-related education. Secure messaging is defined as one that is HIPAA compliant and regulates who has access to the communication as well as how these messages are stored. It includes end-to-end encryption, which prevents anyone but the sender and intended recipient from monitoring the conversation. In end-to-end encryption (E2EE) data is encrypted on the sender's system or device. It travels to its destination in a format that cannot be read or tampered with by an internet service provider (ISP), application service provider, individual hacker, or any other service or person. It is then received by the intended recipient and is decrypted as only the intended recipient can perform this action. This secure messaging process includes sending and receiving messages via chat, email, and through file exchange. EHR systems are being used to facilitate these virtual visits and integrate findings as part of the permanent patient record. Virtual visits incorporate live communications with one's actual care provider.

Telehealth and telemedicine are not the same, although individuals may use these terms interchangeably. Telemedicine uses technology to provide remote patient clinical services. These services may include real-time consultations and interactions, remote monitoring, and reviewing of specific information sent by the patient that can be reviewed by the provider and remotely responded to at a later time. Telehealth encompasses telemedicine services but has an expanded reach that includes nonclinical services such as administrative meetings, continued medical education, and health care provider training.

Fast Health Care Interoperability Resources

Fast Health care Interoperability Resources (FHIR) is a Health Level Seven (HL7) standard that is designed to provide for the exchange of health care information among applications and systems regardless of their underlying architecture. This means that regardless of the way a provider's or health information systems EHR technology stores or represents the data, it will be shared in a standard way. FHIR is designed to be flexible and adaptable. It can allow data sharing in clinical settings and better align with decision support initiatives, which ultimately can improve patient care delivery. This exchange network is open source (publicly accessible and can be accessed, modified, and freely distributed) and advances interoperability.

What is HL7? HL7 is a set of international clinical data standards and messaging formats. These provide a framework for electronic health care information to be managed, integrated, exchanged, and retrieved across various and different organizational health care computer systems. HL7 was developed by Health Level Seven International, a nonprofit health care standards organization, and continues to be maintained by them.

Reference: HealthIT.gov. (2021, June 16). *FHIR fact sheets*. https://www.healthit.gov/topic/standards-technology/standards/fhir-fact-sheets

Chapter Summary

In order for the EHRS to navigate the evolving health care landscape of EHRs, they must be familiar with key informatics concepts. Interoperability, as it relates to the EHR, refers to the ability of different health care systems and applications to seamlessly exchange and use patient health information regardless of their on-premises internal structure or cloud-based designated vendor. Achieving interoperability improves care coordination, health care professional communication, and patient engagement in their care. AI is revolutionizing health care as it promotes health care capabilities for advanced analytics, decision-making, and predictive modeling. Patient-generated health data allows individuals to input data from various sources (e.g., wearable devices, mobile apps, personal health monitoring tools) into their health record that they feel is important to include or correct information they feel is in error with validation. This gives a total patient picture for health care professional intervention. Telehealth technologies enable remote delivery of health care services with virtual consultations, remote monitoring, and telemedicine visits. By recognizing and leveraging these technologies, the EHRS can enhance organizational interoperability and services, and support improved patient outcomes.

10

MEDICAL/BUSINESS TERMINOLOGY AND ABBREVIATIONS

CHAPTER OBJECTIVES

Upon completion of this chapter, the reader will be able to do the following:

1. Discuss the Systematized Nomenclature of Medicine–Clinical Terms.
2. Define basic health care finance terminology.
3. Recognize prefixes and suffixes used in medical terminology.
4. Convey the meaning of some common medical abbreviations and terms.

KEY CHAPTER TERMS

- Systematized Nomenclature of Medicine–Clinical Terms (SNOMED CT)
- Basic health care finance terminologies
- Medical terminologies

Systematized Nomenclature of Medicine–Clinical Terms

Systematized Nomenclature of Medicine–Clinical Terms (SNOMED CT) is a comprehensive multilingual clinical terminology that originated from the Systematic Nomenclature of Pathology

(SNOP) by the College of American Pathologists. Through collaborative development, it meets the needs of a diverse worldwide medical community. As a result, it is accepted as a common global language for health terms in over 50 countries. It facilitates interoperability as it can be mapped to other coding systems (e.g., ICD-11). This nomenclature of medicine is evidence-based and research validated, which gives it a high level of credibility for use. Due to this credibility level, it can be used to consistently and comprehensively represent relevant clinical information. The United States has designated SNOMED CT as the national standard for additional EHR categories and for health information exchange. The U.S. SNOMED CT International Edition is released bi-annually with the current schedule of March and September (https://www.nlm.nih.gov/healthit/snomedct/us_edition.html).

Basic Health Care Finance Terminology

Health care finance includes accounting and fiscal management for a health care organization. These terms generally follow those as defined by corporate and financial institutions. They are not uniquely defined by the health care sector. The following are some **basic health care finance terminologies** that you need to be familiar with.

Definitions

Budget: A plan for company income and expenditures for a designated period (e.g., quarterly, bi-annually, annually). This is important as it designates how a company or entity expects to acquire and use resources for financial profit.

Capital budgeting: The process of analyzing and choosing long-term assets. Technological tools can be used to facilitate this outcome through analysis of cash inflow and outflow for benchmark identification and goal attainment.

Capital investment: The process of acquiring funds or physical assets for the growth of a company or organization. Monies are usually set aside to promote the achievement of future business financial goals and objectives.

Chief financial officer: A person responsible for all organizational financial activities, which can include budgeting, tracking cash flow, expense and income forecasting, financial risk management, and account management.

Contract management: The systematic handling of contracts, which includes negotiating, signing, and monitoring. Efficient control ensures that contracts are current and comply with legal requirements as well as promote the achievement of organizational goals.

Corporation: A company or group that is authorized by a state to act as a single entity with a common goal. It is separate from its owners and recognized by law.

Financial report: A document generated to identify the current financial position of a company or health care organization. This is usually done on a quarterly and/or annual basis.

Financial statement: A document prepared by accountants that identifies the current status of monetary receipts and expenditures of an organization.

Fiscal year: The financial year for a company; any 12-month period. It may or may not follow the standard calendar year.

For-profit: An entity designed to be in business to generate monies for individuals in the company and investors. This type of organization must file taxes each year, along with disclosures, usually through their financial report.

Health insurance: A company or government agency that provides payment of services given by health care entities.

Not-for-profit: An organization that is formed for a specific purpose and does not distribute funds to its members but rather uses them mainly for philanthropic purposes (provision of services to enhance certain components of society; e.g., breast cancer). This type of organization is called a 501c3 or 501c4 (U.S. Internal Revenue Code) as this designation makes it tax exempt.

Partnership: An association of two or more people who come together for business purposes. This formal arrangement allows them to manage and operate a business together, sharing profits as well as liabilities or losses.

Proprietorship: A business owned by a single person. Usually called a sole proprietorship.

Revenue cycle: A set of repetitive business activities, which indicate exchange of goods or services for payment (e.g., order for services, customer service recognition of order, order shipped, billing for order sent, funds received, next order, etc.).

Risk management: The process of identifying, assessing, controlling, and minimizing uncertainties (expenditures) in a business that can reduce capital or earnings. This can determine the success of a company.

Stakeholder: An individual who has an interest in a designated business. They work to ensure business success through a positive return on investment for the company.

Medical Terminology

Health care can have its own language when it comes to medical terms as well as prefixes and suffixes. It is important for the EHRS to have a basic understanding of these in order to accurately document information in the system. This will also promote your understanding when communicating with health care providers. This list is not all inclusive but does contain some basic medical terminologies, prefixes, suffixes, common medical abbreviations, with definitions of common terms for illnesses and medical conditions, in alphabetical order.

Definitions

Adverse drug event: Complications or side effects from a specific drug administered to a patient.

Adverse event: An event in health care that occurs and causes patient harm that resulted from treatment or care given.

Anatomy: Study of the structure and organization of living organisms, including humans*.

CPT codes: A system of codes used to identify and classify medical procedures and services*.

Diagnosis: Identification of a specific condition or disease based on symptoms, medical history, and diagnostic tests*.

Electronic prescribing (eRx): A process of electronically prescribing medications to a patient*.

Formulary: A list of medications, also called a drug list, covered by a prescription plan or insurance plan offering prescription benefits. This list usually identifies medications that are identified as the best, least expensive, or most economical for condition treatment. This list includes generic and brand names for medication.

Health insurance: A system of coverage that pays for medical expenses*.

HIPAA: A federal law that regulates the privacy and security of patient health information*.

ICD-11 codes: System of codes (11th edition) used to identify and classify diseases and medical conditions. It is a basis for medical reimbursement.

Lab values: Measurements of various substances in the body, such as blood glucose levels or cholesterol levels*.

Medicare Part A: Hospital insurance plan that helps cover hospital care, nursing facility care, hospice care, and home health care.

Medicare Part B: Medical insurance that helps cover services from physicians and other health care providers, outpatient care, durable medical equipment, preventive services, outpatient, and home health care.

Medicare Part C: Medicare Advantage plan, which is a Medicare-approved plan from a private company that offers an alternative to the original Medicare plan for health and drug coverage.

Medicare Part D: Voluntary Medicare drug benefit plan paid by the patient.

Medical history: A record of a patient's past and present medical conditions, treatments, and medications*.

Medications: Drugs prescribed to treat or prevent medical conditions or manage symptoms*.

National Council for Prescription Drug Program (NCPDP): A nonprofit organization that (a) develops standards for product labeling, dosing instructions, and patient communication to minimize patient dosing errors; (b) facilitates real-time information exchange for prescribing, dispensing, monitoring, managing and payments; (c) develops standards for product labeling, medication dosing instructions, and communication with patients to reduce dosing errors; (d) provides tools for accurate data collection and mitigation of fraud, waste, and abuse (FWA); and (e) collects pharmacy count data based on unique licensed pharmacy identifiers.

Notice of privacy: Document from a health care provider or health plan shared with care recipients that disclose privacy rights and how the provider or plan might use and share personal health information.

Pathology: Study of diseases and the effects they have on the body*.

Physiology: Study of how living organisms function and operate*.

Point of Care: Setting where a health care provider administers care and makes decisions related to that care delivery.

Procedures: Medical interventions or treatments, such as surgeries, imaging tests, or laboratory tests*.

Prognosis: A predicted course and outcome of a disease or condition*.

United Medical Language System (UMLS): A set of files and software organized by concept that bring together several health and biomedical vocabularies to promote interoperability between computer systems.

- Metathesaurus: A large biomedical thesaurus that is the largest component of the UMLS.

Vital signs: Measurements of a patient's basic body functions, such as blood pressure, heart rate, respiratory rate, and body temperature*.

*OpenAI. (2023). ChatGPT (Mar 14 version) [Large language model]. https://chat.openai.com/chat

Prefixes and Suffixes

Prefix	Meaning	Suffix	Meaning
a-	Absence of	-algia	Pain
Ab-	Away from	-emia	Blood condition
Ad-	Towards	-itis	Inflammation
Anti-	Against	-meter	Measuring instrument
Contra-	Against	-metry	Process of measuring
Dextr(o)-	Right; on the right side	-paresis	Slight paralysis
Digit-	Finger	-pathy	Disease; disorder
Epi-	Outside of	-penia	Deficiency
Gastro-	Stomach	-phage, -phagia	Eating or ingestion condition
Hema/hemo-	Blood	-plasty	Surgical repair
Hyper-	Above normal	-plegia	Paralysis
Hypo-	Below normal	-rrhagia	discharge
Infra-	Beneath; below	-rrhea	discharge
Inter-	Between	-rrhexis	rupture
Intra-	Within	-scope	Instrument for viewing
Leuk(o)-	White	-scopy	Use of viewing instrument
Macro/mega-	Large	-stomy	Creation of an opening
Meso-	Middle	-tome	Cutting instrument
Micro-	Small	-tomy	Cutting operation
Normo-	Normal		
Ossi-	Bone		
Peri-	Around		
Phago-	Eating; devouring		
Pharmaco-	Drug; medication		

(*Continued*)

Prefix	Meaning	Suffix	Meaning
Phleb(o)	Blood		
Post-	Behind; after		
Pre-	Before; in front		
Presby(o)	Old age		
Proct(o)	Anus; rectum		
Pyo-	Pus		
Pyro-	Fever		
Quadr(i)	Four		
Retro-	Backward; behind		
Rhin-	Reference to nose		
Sub-	Under; beneath		
Super-	Above		
Supra-	Above		
Tachy-	Fast		
Thrombo-	Blood clotting		
Uni-	One		
Uro-	Urinary system		
Urin-	Urine		
Uter(o)	Uterus or womb		
Vasculo	Blood vessel		
Viscer(o)	Internal organs		

Some Common Medical Abbreviations

See https://www.asha.org/practice-portal/professional-issues/documentation-in-health-care/common-medical-abbreviations/.

Abbreviation	Meaning
A	
AAROM	Active Assistive Range of Motion
ABG	Arterial blood gases
a.c.	Before meals

Abbreviation	Meaning
A/C	Assist control
ADL	Activities of daily living
A Fib	Atrial fibrillation (abnormal heart rhythm)
AKA	Above-knee amputation
A & O	Alert and oriented
AMA	Against medical advice
A/P	Anterior-posterior
ASAP	As soon as possible
B	
bid	Twice a day
Bilat	Bilateral
BKA	Below-knee amputation
BMR	Basal metabolic rate
BP	Blood pressure
BR	Bedrest
BS	Breath sounds / bowel sounds (based on part of body referenced)
Bx	Biopsy
C	
$\bar{c}$	With
C	Celsius
C1, C2, etc.	Cervical vertebrae by number
CA	Cancer
CABG	Coronary artery bypass graft
CAD	Coronary artery disease
Cal	Calorie
Cath	Catheter
CBC	Complete blood count
CC	Chief complaint
CHF	Congestive heart failure
CCU	Coronary care unit
CNA	Certified nursing assistant
CNS	Central nervous system
c/o	Complains of

(Continued)

Abbreviation	Meaning
Cont	Continued
COPD	Chronic obstructive pulmonary disease
CPAP	Continuous positive airway pressure
CPR	Cardiopulmonary resuscitation
CRF	Chronic renal failure
CRNP	Certified registered nurse practitioner
CT	Computerized tomography
CV	Cardiovascular
CSF	Cerebrospinal fluid
CVA	Cerebral vascular accident
CXR	Chest X-ray
D	
d/c	Discontinue
DC	Discharge
DM	Diabetes mellitus
DNKA	Did not keep appointment
DNR	Do not resuscitate
DOA	Dead on arrival
DOB	Date of birth
d/t	Due to
Dx	Diagnosis
E	
ECG/EKG	Electrocardiogram
ED	Emergency department
EEG	Electroencephalogram
EENT	Eyes, ears, nose, throat
ENT	Ears, nose, throat
ER	Emergency room
ETOH	Ethanol/alcohol
Exam	Examination
Ext	External, exterior
F	
F	Fahrenheit
FH	Family history

Abbreviation	Meaning
Fib	Fibrillation
Fl, fld	Fluid
FOB	Foot of bed
f/u	Follow-up
FWB	Full weight bearing
Fx	Fracture
G	
GB	Gallbladder
GCS	Glascow coma scale
GERD	Gastroesophageal reflux disease
Gen	General
Gest.	Gestation
GI	Gastrointestinal
Gluc	Glucose
GP	General practitioner
GSW	Gunshot wound
GTT	Glucose tolerance test
GYN	Gynecology
H	
h	Hour
H/A	Headache
Hb	Heart block
HBP	High blood pressure
HEENT	Head, eyes, ears, nose, throat
H2O	Water
h/o	History of
HOB	Head of bed
H&P	History and physical
HR	Heart rate
HTN	Hypertension
HVD	Hypertensive vascular disease
Hx	History
I	
ICP	Intracranial pressure

(Continued)

Abbreviation	Meaning
ICU	Intensive care unit
Int.	Internal
I&O	Intake and output
IPPB	Intermittent positive pressure breathing
IV	Intravascular
K	
K	Potassium
L	
L	Left, liter, lower, lumbar (based on reference)
L2, L3, etc.	Lumbar vertebrae by number
Lab	Laboratory
Lac	Laceration
Lat	Lateral
LBW	Low birth weight
LE	Lower extremity
Liq	Liquid
LOC	Level of consciousness
LOS	Length of stay
LP	Lumbar puncture
LPN	Licensed practical nurse
LUE	Left upper extremity
L&W	Living and well
M	
m, M	Married, male, mother, murmur, meter, mass, molar (based on reference)
Max.	Maximum, maxillary
MBC	Maximum breathing capacity
MD	Muscular dystrophy (disease)
MD	Medical doctor (health care provider)
Med.	Medicine
Mets.	Metastasis
MI	Myocardial infarction
Min	Minute

Abbreviation	Meaning
MICU	Medical intensive care unit
Mod	Moderate
MRI	Magnetic resonance imaging
MRSA	Methicillin-resistant *Staphylococcus aureus*
MVA	Motor vehicle accident
N	
Na	Sodium
NaCl	Sodium chloride
NAD	No abnormality detected / no apparent distress
Neg	Negative
Neuro	Neurology
NG	Nasogastric
NIC	Neonatal intensive care unit
NKA	No known allergies
NPO	Nothing per os (nothing by mouth)
NST	Nonstress test
N&V	Nausea and vomiting
N&W	Normal and well
NWB	Nonweight bearing
NYD	Not yet diagnosed
O	
O	Oral
O_2	Oxygen
O_2 sat.	Oxygen saturation
OA	Osteoarthritis
OB	Obstetrics
OB/GYN	Obstetrics and gynecology
Obs	Observation
OBS	Organic brain syndrome
Oint	Ointment
O.M.	Otitis media
OOB	Out of bed
OTC	Over the counter (medication)

(*Continued*)

Abbreviation	Meaning
OR	Operating room
P	
PA	Physician's assistant
PACU	Post anesthesia care unit
Palp	Palpate, palpated, palpation
PA view	Posterior-anterior view on X-ray
P.C.	After meals
PE	Physical examination
Ped	Pediatrics
PEEP	Positive end expiratory pressure
PET	Positron emission tomography
PI	Present illness
P.M.	Afternoon
P.O.	Per os (by mouth)
Postop	Postoperative (after surgery)
PRN	As often as needed
Pt.	Patient
PT	Physical therapy
PVD	Peripheral vascular disease
Q	
q	Every
QD/qd	Every day
QID/qid	Four times a day
R	
RA	Rheumatoid arthritis
RBC/rbc	Red blood cells
Rehab	Rehabilitation
Resp	Respiratory
RLE	Right lower extremity
RN	Registered nurse
ROM	Range of motion
ROS	Review of systems
Rt	Right

Abbreviation	Meaning
RUE	Right upper extremity
Rx	Prescription
S	
s	Without
SCD	Sudden cardiac death
SH	Social history
SICU	Surgical intensive care unit
SIDS	Sudden infant death syndrome
SL	Sublingual (under the tongue)
SOB	Shortness of breath
S/S	Signs and symptoms
Stat	Immediately
STD	Sexually transmitted disease
Subq	Subcutaneous
Sx	Symptoms
Syst	Systolic
T	
T	Temperature
Tab	Tablet
Temp	Temperature
THR	Total hip replacement
TIA	Transient ischemic attack
TPR	Temperature, pulse, respiration
Trach	Tracheostomy
Tx	Treatment
U	
U/A	Urinalysis
Unilat	Unilateral
URI	Upper respiratory infection
UTI	Urinary tract infection
V	
VD	Venereal disease
Vent	Ventilator

(Continued)

Abbreviation	Meaning
Vit	Vitamin
V.S./VS	Vital signs
W	
W/C	Wheelchair
w/n	Within
WNL	Within normal limits
wt.	Weight
X	
x	Times
Y	
Yrs.	Years

Some Common Terms, Illnesses and Medical Conditions

Term	Definition
Acute	A medical condition that starts quickly.
Angina	Chest pain that comes and goes (intermittent) caused by not enough blood flow to the heart muscle.
Allergy	An overaction of the body's immune system to something in the environment or a medication that can cause a reaction from hives to difficulty breathing or even death.
Alzheimer's disease	A brain disorder that gets worse and cannot be reversed, which results in memory loss, the ability to speak, and the ability to take care of oneself.
Arthritis	Inflammation of a joint that causes pain and reduces the ability to move it.
Asthma	A condition of the lungs that causes difficulty breathing, coughing, and wheezing that occurs over a prolonged period of time (usually caused by increased activity or contact with something the person is allergic to).
Benign	A tumor that is not cancerous.
Cellulitis	An infection of a deep layer of the skin.

Term	Definition
Chlamydia	An infection of the vagina, penis, or rectum caused by bacteria; can be sexually transmitted.
Chronic	A condition that is continuous over an extended period of time.
Congenital	Something that occurs from birth.
Dehydration	A condition that occurs when the body loses too much water and other fluids; can occur from excessive sweating, diarrhea, or failure to drink enough water.
Depression	A mental state in which a person has a poor outlook on life.
Diabetes	A chronic disease that occurs when the pancreas (a body organ) does not produce enough insulin or when the body cannot efficiently use the insulin produced.
Dysphagia	Difficulty swallowing.
Edema	Swelling caused by retention of fluid in the body; can occur in arms legs or over the entire body.
Embolism	A blockage in the circulatory system caused by a foreign material, usually blood components (platelets, proteins, and cells stick together; called a blood clot), but can be caused by fat or air.
Epilepsy	A condition in which brain activity is abnormal, which can cause seizures or episodes of unusual behavior, sensations, and sometimes loss of what an individual is doing or knowledge of what is going on around them.
Febrile	An abnormally high body temperature.
Fracture	A crack or broken bone in the body.
Gout	A painful condition of the joints where crystals form inside and around them.
Hepatitis	Inflammation of the liver.
Human Immunodeficiency Virus	Often referred to as HIV. A virus that attacks the body's immune system that can lead to AIDS (Acquired Immunodeficiency Syndrome).
Hypertension	High blood pressure.

(Continued)

Term	Definition
Hypotension	Low blood pressure.
Influenza	A contagious illness of the respiratory (breathing) system caused by the influenza virus. Commonly called the flu and can affect the nose and throat in addition to the lungs.
Intravenous	A medication or fluid given directly in a vein.
Lesion	Injury to the skin (e.g., sore).
Malignant	A growth or tumor that is cancerous and has the ability to spread to other body parts.
Migraine	A moderate to severe head pain that can be throbbing or pulsing.
Myocardial infarction	A heart attack caused by poor blood supply to the heart, where some of the muscle is injured or dies due to lack of oxygen carried in the blood.
Osteoporosis	A condition that occurs when the body does not replenish bone as fast as it is normally being broken down and results in a porous bone that is easier to break.
Pleurisy	An infection of the tissue layer that surrounds the lungs.
Pneumonia	An infection in lobes of one or both lungs.
Remission	A disease that has stopped progressing.
Sepsis	Infection of the body or part of the body.
Stroke	Also sometimes called a "brain attack" that results from a blocked artery or a ruptured artery in the brain.
Thrombosis/ thrombus	A blood clot in blood circulation.
Tinnitus	Abnormal sounds that originate from inside the body often called "ringing in the ear(s)" but can be a buzzing, hissing humming, or whistling sound.
Ulcer	An open sore, wound, or break in the external skin on the body or on the surface of an organ inside of the body.
Urticaria	Medical term for "hives" or "welts" that occur from an allergic response.

Chapter Summary

Health care has its own language, and understanding this language promotes effective communication and verification of documentation. SNOMED CT is a comprehensive and multilingual clinical terminology system. It promotes standardization of clinical concepts and facilitates interoperability across health care settings. The EHRS must know basic health care terms, such as the difference between a financial report and financial statement, as well as medical terminology, such as adverse event, pathology, point of care, and so on. The EHRS must be able to understand common prefixes and suffixes as they provide clues to the meaning of the medical term. By having the ability to define SNOMED CT, understand basic health care finance terminology, recognize medical prefixes and suffixes, and identify common medical abbreviations, the EHRS can enhance their proficiency in medical terminology and finance, and effectively communicate both verbally and in writing.

11

EHRS CERTIFICATION TEST PLAN SPECIFIC INFORMATION

CHAPTER OBJECTIVES

Upon completion of this chapter, the reader will be able to do the following:

1. Summarize EHRS examination components.
2. Identify three ways to prepare for the Certified Electronic Health Records Specialist examination.
3. Develop a plan for success for the CEHRS examination.
4. Recall success requirements for the CEHRS examination.
5. Recognize domains and sub-domains for the CEHRS examination.

Certification test plan detailed information is in this chapter. The following sections are specifically organized to address components from the EHRS certification examination test plan.

Nonclinical Operations (28% of Exam; 28 Items)

Verify patient identifiers before documenting in the EHR to ensure information is recorded in the correct chart.

The EHR specialist verifies patient information. This verification process is crucial to perform prior to documenting in the EHR to ensure that accurate information is in the correct patient chart.

The following are some of the common identification methods used prior to documentation in the EHR; by verifying patient identification before documentation, the EHR specialist can help to prevent errors and ensure that patient data is complete and accurate.

- Verbal verification: Ask the patient to state their full name and date of birth. This is to be confirmed by comparison to information in the EHR.
- Visual verification: Check the patient's identification bracelet. This is to be confirmed by comparison to information in the EHR.
- Biometric verification: Use fingerprint, eye, or facial recognition via a software program. This is to be verified through a 'match' to information already in the system.
- Second-person verification: Have a second health care provider validate identify. This validation can be done prior to other forms of verification. This is not to be the only form of verification used for comparison to information in the system.

Collect, record, and continuously update patient information (e.g., demographic information, clinical data, coverages/financial/insurance, guarantors, patient preferences).

The key to accuracy is a combination of collecting, recording, and continuously updating patient information. Patient demographic information must be verified, clinical data must be updated with interventions, patient preferences clarified, and coverage information maintained current (financial responsibility of patient versus insurance or guarantors).

The following responsibilities of the EHR specialist fall under this category:

- Collect patient information.
- Enter information into the patient EHR.
- Update patient information as necessary to keep current.
- Verify information accuracy.
- Ensure patient privacy.

Generate encounter documentation (e.g., admission/face sheet, labels, armbands).

On admission all individuals will be entered into the health record system and identified using an armband with information generated for use by the care provider. The admission/face sheet is generated by computer based on data retrieval at the time. Labels may also be generated that accompany the admission sheet to be used for patient identification related to procedures, laboratory specimen labeling, medication administration, and procedure validation. Some intake armbands are color coded to identify patients at risk (e.g., fall risk). The intake is essential as it not only allows for retrieval of information but allows for validation of this information by the patient or family. The armband is securely placed on the patient at this initial entry meeting and is the one used throughout the entire care provision stay. It often includes the individual's name, specific patient identification number (permanent patient identifier), and scanning barcode and may include allergies as well as date of birth.

Retrieve patient information from internal databases (e.g., provider database, financial database) to integrate into a patient's EHR.

Patient data can be partitioned in several independent databases that may require retrieval and summarization (compilation and placement into the current patient EHR). It is imperative that the specialist be familiar with the types of databases available in the working institution or clinic and be able to access and obtain correct information for inclusion into the record for currency and implementation of accurate care based on this information. Provider databases may include the following:

- Health record data such as patient demographic information, diagnoses, treatment modalities, prescribed and administered medications, and laboratory tests obtained.
- Claims data, which can include inpatient, outpatient, pharmaceutical, and enrollment information for patients.
- Financial data, which may include organizational assets, expenses, revenues, and liabilities.
- Patient or disease registries, which maintain clinical information related to tracking key data for diseases such as cancer, diabetes, heart disease, and so on.

Acquire patient data from external sources (e.g., diagnostic laboratories, ancillary facilities, other healthcare providers, other EHR systems).

There are several ways to obtain data from external sources. These allow for retrieval of information across organizations and improve collaboration. It can also improve patient care as it allows for information access that may be relevant to the current hospitalization or care delivery intent.

- Extract, transform, and load (ETL): This is a basic level for data retrieval. This data is usually obtained at specifically identified regular intervals. Data from one system is retrieved (extracted), changed to another form or appearance (transformed), and placed in the new source (loaded).
- Application Programming Interface (API): The API is a set of defined rules that allow communication between different applications. It is an intermediary layer that delivers a request from one application to another. This allows for data transfer between systems, which allows companies to open their data applications to other companies.
- Fast Health care Interoperability Resources (FHIR): The FHIR is an exchange framework to advance interoperability. In addition to data exchange specifications, FHIR capabilities include infrastructure, administrative, and clinical capabilities.

Import information into the EHR from integrated devices (e.g., scanners, fax machines, e-signature pads, cameras).

There is an increasing demand for information integration from various sources. Many EHRs now have the capability to automatically integrate retrieved information directly from equipment such as data-receiving devices (scanners, fax machines, e-signature pads, cameras). These EHRs can also import information such as vital signs from medical devices (vital sign retrieval hardware machines) and even intravenous infusion pumps (smart pumps). If these are not built into the EHR system, it will require that manual input be completed. This is a time-sensitive requirement and must be done daily in order to maintain EHR currency. Fax machines and scanners are still in use for transmission of EHRs due to the lack of interoperability among various systems. Faxing information may require a coversheet that includes a checklist of specific items and an audit log (name of sender, organization represented, date, time, recipient name, recipient phone number, and contact information for sender). It is also imperative to be familiar with policies for transport of information among devices and even across state lines.

Maintain inventory of EHR-related hardware (e.g., e-signature pads, cameras, tablets, mobile devices).

Inventory is important to identify company assets. This should be maintained in a current status for purchases and disposals. A generalized audit is usually done on an annual basis. Inventory involves identifying all hardware owned, rented, or leased with key information related to specific identification numbers given by the organization for inventory purposes, date of entry into the system, type of acquisition (purchase, rent or lease), date for replacement, if there is such a schedule and warranty information (warranty time-frame, especially identification of the expiration date). Inventory should also include the location of equipment, which is critical for onsite walk-around validation. Some inventories can also include asset depreciation for the reduction in asset value over time and asset disposal to identify when and how a piece of equipment was removed from service. Any information related to maintenance agreements should be retained and schedules kept, ensuring equipment is in the best possible condition.

Coordinate patient flow within the facility (e.g., scheduling, patient registration and verification, check-in/check-out, patient referrals).

Management of patient flow allows for improved patient satisfaction and higher employee proficiency. In order to accomplish the best facility flow, scheduling must be based on algorithms used for timing of patient appointments and allowances for potential "no shows," which may be as high as 10% based on facility data. Effective coordination relies on decision-making tools, resource monitoring, internal systems, and medical care resources.

Provide initial and ongoing end user training of EHR software to maintain competency (e.g., for new hires, upgrades, and deployments).

Any part of a job is staying up-to-date on new innovations and applications relevant to one's responsibilities. In order to provide initial and ongoing end user training, the EHR specialist must maintain knowledge and expertise in EHR software and hardware being used by the organization. This allows all organizational end users to stay up-to-date on current and new features in systems used for patient record intake and maintenance. The EHR specialist must identify employee computer skills essential to maintain and provide training and updates to these systems minimally on an annual basis for current employees. The specialist must work with administration and other technology specialists in the organization to create a training plan and identify essential skills necessary for employees to effectively interact with the EHR system. The specialist will not only provide initial training and updates but also provide intermittent support throughout the term of employment for staff.

Share information about updates to EHR software and the implications for workflow.

Updates to EHR software are essential to the effective workflow in an organization. Outdated software may not only pose a threat to security but may also cause a loss of essential information retrieval. The flow of clinician workflow can also be negatively affected by outdated EHR software. Updates may also require workflow redesign. Efficient redesign can enhance the quality of health care delivery, provide patient safety, and improve care coordination. Working with the software vendor to make choices that will effectively and efficiently promote organizational workflow is also important.

Identify data discrepancies within and among multiple EHRs, practice management systems, and other software systems.

Data is only as good as the input system or individual. Discrepancies can occur in data among practice management systems and the multiple EHR systems required for interaction in order to deliver effective client care. Many organizations will have data governance frameworks that are designed to ensure that data is accurate, complete, and consistent across multiple software systems. Errors caused by configuration and usability issues can result in patient safety situations such as errors in medication dose timing. Data quality issues are magnified when data source systems are not kept synchronized. Data errors must be corrected, and duplicate entries must be identified and corrected in a timely and comprehensive fashion. An EHR plan for downtime readiness and recovery will serve to ensure meaningful and enhanced computer system management.

Report or reconcile data discrepancies within and among multiple EHRs, practice management systems, and other software systems.

Reporting and reconciling data discrepancies, inconsistencies, and errors within and among systems is a critical responsibility of the EHR specialist. This is crucial in order to maintain accurate data. This is done through data audits and analyses at scheduled and intermittent times based on the amount of information, organizational need, and regulatory requirements. This facilitates interoperability and promotes prompt reconciliation. The specialist must enforce standardized coding and terminology in and among systems to ensure consistency. This can be done by using terminologies such as SNOMED and ICD codes. If there is an error logging and notification system, addressing these entries allows for prompt notification, when required, based on internal and regulatory policies and procedures. Being proactive about reporting and reconciliation can serve to improve organizational effectiveness.

Provide support to patients regarding their use of patient portals (e.g., basic introduction, explain utility, grant access, navigation help).

The patient portal is an online platform for patients to access their electronic health record as well as review reports and communicate with their health care provider. The EHR specialist offers patient support with portal access through education and training to promote an understanding of what can and cannot be done in the portal. Many portals offer the patient an opportunity to read and review their records, laboratory and radiology reports, and securely communicate with their provider for concerns or getting medications refilled. Education can be done on an on-demand basis through written information that is available in electronic or hand-out format or through online videos. The EHR specialist can also assist with trouble shooting for patients who may have difficulty registering, accessing, or engaging with the system. Patient information access may be available through a desktop software program or a mobile application.

Clinical Operations (32% of Exam; 32 Items)

Develop clinical templates for data capture (e.g., by diagnosis, by procedure, by practice).

Clinical templates promote standardization of data entry for retrieval. Software systems often come with generic templates, but these must be revised to capture specific organization information. Standardizing data entry through the use of templates improves documentation efficiency, saving clinical time required for information input, and ensures that relevant information is captured and input is standardized for report retrieval. Clinical templates should use structured data fields and dropdown menus whenever possible. This allows for ease of data entry and avoids free text fields that allow for varying terms to be used by providers for the same procedure or activity. Templates with structured data fields maintain consistency and enhance data quality retrieval. The use of template alerts and reminders through identification of required fields prior to proceeding to another screen also promotes record completion.

Securely transmit and exchange patient data internally and externally (e.g., to pharmacies, other healthcare providers, other agencies) for research, analytics, and continuity of care.

Security of transmission and exchange of patient data is managed through a strong security network infrastructure. This is accomplished through encryption protocols. An encryption protocol is a fundamental aspect of cybersecurity that uses a set of rules or algorithms that change it into a coded, unreadable format until it is received by the appropriate designee with the key for decoding (decryption key). Some of the more common encryption protocols used in the health care industry are as follows:

- Hypertext Transfer Protocol Secure (HTTPS) is the secure version of HTTP. This is the primary protocol used to send data between a web browser and a website. This encrypts communications and increases security for sites such as banks or health care provider organization information. HTTPS prevents websites from having their information sent out in a way that can be easily viewed by anyone. HTTPS is encrypted information that increases data transfer security. This is indicated by the use of an S in the uniform resource locater (URL) bar after HTTP, which means that the site is using a Secure Sockets Layer (SSL) certificate.

- A Secure Sockets Layer (SSL) ensures privacy, authentication, and integrity by creating an authentication channel between internet devices. Using this encryption protocol means that information can be securely shared. SSL eventually evolved into Transport Layer Security (TLS). SSL is the predecessor of TLS, and the terms are often interchanged due to their direct relationship and purpose. TLS and SSL can have certificates (SSL/TLS Certificate), which is a digital object that allows a system to validate, identify, and establish an encrypted network connection. These are purchased from a certificate authority and identify and validate the domain owner and the server's public key.
- Advanced Encryption Standard (AES) 256 is a symmetric encryption algorithm that uses a 256-bit key for conversion of plain text or data to a block cipher. The block cipher is a fixed block size that is processed through a series of transformations to create encrypted output. It uses the same key for encryption and decryption, and this key is 256 bits long in this algorithm, which equates to a number with 77 digits, which makes it very secure.

Review and monitor clinical documentation to ensure completeness and accuracy (e.g., self-review, peer-to-peer).

The EHR specialist must verify that all documentation is complete and accurate—their own and that of employees working for the organization. Self-review requires that the specialist randomly retrieves information at various intervals to verify its accuracy, clarity, consistency, and completeness across databases. The peer-to-peer review requires that the specialist collaborate with their peers, which can include other organizational specialists or colleagues. This collaborative effort allows for mutual reviews of each other's documentation for accuracy, clarity, consistency, and completeness. All reviews must be done while adhering to organizational and regulatory requirements.

Provide point-of-care EHR support (e.g., at-the-elbow, remote) for clinical documentation.

- At-the-elbow point-of-care support is assisting health care workers directly on their units or at their specific organizational workstations. During these encounters, the EHR specialist can directly review and monitor processes for employee access to patient records and the direct input of clinical data to ensure compliance. This can allow face-to-face assistance with database access, interface navigation, input of patient information, and access to various components of the patient EHR. This type of interaction often occurs when employees require onsite troubleshooting for issues related to specific EHR components.
- Remote point-of-care support is when the EHR specialist assists health care workers from a distance through electronic means. Contact is made through video conferencing, chat, or phone. The employee can be onsite or working remotely from another location. These encounters assist with database access, interface navigation, input of patient information, and access to various components of the patient EHR. This type of interaction often occurs when employees require troubleshooting from offsite locations for issues related to specific EHR components.

Input real-time clinical data into the EHR.

Real time is the actual time of an occurrence or when an event occurs. This type of data is available to the user or others within milliseconds or microseconds—virtually immediately following input by an individual. By recording health care data when it happens, the record is maintained in a current state, and there can be quicker turnaround time for activities that are ordered and their results, which leads to faster implementation. This can reduce repetitive documentation and better promote compliance. By reducing repetitive entries, this can reduce workload. The critically important component for real-time data entry is that this data must be accurate upon input.

Document patient historic clinical data in the EHR (e.g., medications, immunizations, surgeries).

Documenting the patient historic clinical data in the EHR requires that there is validation for past illnesses and treatments, surgeries with outcomes, immunizations received, laboratory and radiological results, past health encounters for wellness checks, and so forth. Completeness of the past health record is important for access of accurate information and current and future effective patient care management. The EHR specialist must be familiar with various components of the record such as the computerized provider order entry (CPOE) system where orders are input by the provider and the location of record components (specifically how to access the various databases for accurate and correct data entry). This is necessary for validation of historical clinical data in the correct area of the EHR.

Provide support for computerized provider order entry (CPOE).

The EHR specialist provides support to individuals and the organization as a whole related to the computerized provider order entry (CPOE) system. The CPOE can also be referred to as the computerized provider order management (CPOM) system since this system does more than just allow for input of orders. The system not only accepts orders but can forward them to the appropriate department for implementation. This system can allow prescriptions to be sent directly to a patient's pharmacy, whether it is inside or outside of the organization. Laboratory and radiological orders can be sent directly to the respective department. These systems often include decision support tools, which can flag medication interactions and even procedures requiring insurance pre-authorization. This allows for expedited care management, improved insurance reimbursement, and reduced errors such as medication errors.

Locate and provide patient education materials available within the EHR.

Patient education materials need to be specific, and the EHR specialist uses the patient's diagnoses, problem list, medication list, and laboratory results to navigate the system and locate designated information specific to these areas for patient education. An order set can be designed that correlates specific patient problems or situations to identified information within the organizational system or retrieved from resources of other companies and entities. An order set is a bundle of specific information based on a patient's condition or other identified piece of data. These predesigned sets deliver information based on this identified patient's condition or identified piece of data but may not take other variables into account, such as patient age, multiple diagnoses, and so on. Some EHR systems identify specific patient education resources through logic built into the system that uses several pieces of patient information to suggest educational material. Information identified through logic can use an algorithm of several patient characteristics inclusive of demographic information and clinical information to identify appropriate educational material, which is more tailored to the patient.

Navigate the EHR system to retrieve requested patient data.

The EHR specialist must be familiar with the EHR interface to know how to retrieve requested data as well as the policies and procedures related to retrieval of this data. Keeping informed and up-to-date on system components and changes are mandatory pieces to proficiency for data retrieval. System navigation can occur through the use of navigation tabs or menus in the system. Advanced searches and system filters can also assist in locating specifically requested information. From the user authentication (specific identification) for log-in for data retrieval to securely logging out of the system, security protocols must be adhered to in order to prevent unauthorized access.

Revenue Cycle/Finance (15% of Exam; 15 Items)

Find codes in databases (e.g., International Statistical Classification of Diseases and Related Health Problems [ICD], Current Procedural Terminology [CPT], and Healthcare Common Procedure Coding System [HCPCS]).

The EHR specialist can use tools integrated into the EHR database or external components of the database to find codes for correct and accurate identification for provider care activities. Some EHRs have built-in code search capability, which allows for key word searching within the EHR system to retrieve specific codes desired.

Lookup can also be done using drop-down menus or picklists. Some EHRs directly communicate with external sources for current information. Using electronic features like favorites and pre-identified smart phrases, which can be built into the system, can also expedite searches and allow for quick retrieval of a code database. Manual searches can be done using hardcopy or electronic copies of codebooks or manuals such as ICD-11, CPT, or HCPCS, but these can be more time-consuming.

Navigate the EHR to create a superbill, encounter forms, fee slips, or charge forms.

Superbills, encounter forms, fee slips, or charge forms are generated through specific functions within the EHR. Automated claims creation and management may be part of the EHR system, which allows retrieval of specific codes and activities for billing purposes and form completion.

- A superbill is generally used for out-of-network providers in that the patient has to pay upfront for specific services and request this statement for submission to be reimbursed for all or portions of the services received. This is a detailed listing of services received that the patient, or a third party used by the patient, then submits to an insurance company for reimbursement consideration. This is the receipt of verification of services, so it must be accurate with correct codes, diagnoses, and so forth needed for insurance reimbursement identification and consideration. This bill type can also be called a fee slip, charge form, charge slip, or fee ticket.
- An encounter form verifies an interaction between a patient and health care provider. These may occur within a hospital (called hospital encounter) or health care office (called office visit). Encounters may be done to assess a patient's health status (e.g., wellness check, follow-up visit, etc.) or provide specific services (e.g., address a chief complaint). This documented interaction can occur in various forms (face-to-face, telephone, telehealth), which can be identified in the EHR as a specific clinical encounter type for selection. These forms may also be referred to as superbills.

Enter the diagnosis and procedure codes billing information (e.g., from a superbill) into the EHR system for claims processing.

The ideal EHR system should be able to generate a medical claim from the superbill, which would include diagnoses and procedure codes. The bill can also be generated from barcodes or scanning devices used by care providers to place components into the system as used for or administered to a given patient and thus be capable of retrieving this information for patient billing. Claims processing will require that the EHR specialist review claims for accuracy and completeness. This must be compared against the plan to verify coverage of services received or that if pre-authorization was required, it was obtained. Forwarding to the correct agency is also required. Some organizations use a clearinghouse for scrubbing, standardizing, and screening of claims prior to being sent to the payor.

Verify that all diagnoses and procedural descriptions for reimbursement are accurately documented in the EHR.

Verifying diagnoses and procedural descriptions for reimbursement in the EHR are a requirement for accurate reimbursement. Using EHR features, the specialist can ensure that medical codes (numbers assigned to specific tasks, services, or procedures), such as the ICD-11 for diagnoses and CPT or HCPCS, for procedures are accurately assigned. Audits should be performed as scheduled or when necessary to validate accuracy. Multiple code types can be used in patient EHRs.

- The ICD-11, for diagnoses, is a global system of medical coding. It allows for classifying diseases, health conditions, and various medical procedures. Each ICD-11 code is linked to a specific diagnosis or medical condition. This allows ICD-11 to promote systematic organization for health information, which facilitates office billing and provider reimbursement for care delivery as well as tracking statistics for public health. Use of this code ensures consistency in communication across health care organizations and billing components.
- CPT codes are used to standardize descriptions for medical, surgical, and diagnostic services and procedures. These codes are created, updated, and maintained by the American Medical Association (AMA). These are the various types of CPT codes:
    - Category I: Identifies codes for procedures or services.

    - Category II: Identifies supplemental or tracking codes for performance measures and quality of care (optional and not required for reimbursement).
    - Category III: Temporary codes for developing new technology, procedures, and services. These codes can be used for things that do not meet Category I for reimbursement consideration.
    - Proprietary Laboratory Analyses (PLA): These codes can be used to add more detailed and specific descriptors for laboratories or manufacturers. These codes include Advanced Diagnostic Laboratory Tests (ADLTs) and Clinical Diagnostic Laboratory Tests (CDLTs). An example of a test in this category could be a Genomic Sequencing Procedure (GSP).
- The Healthcare Common Procedure Coding System (HCPCS) (pronounced "hick-picks") for procedures is a set of health care procedure codes used to submit claims for reimbursement to Medicare and health insurances. They cover a variety of services, supplies, and procedures and allow for consistency in reporting, which promotes accurate communication and reimbursement. There are two divisions or subsystems, which are HCPCS level I and HCPCS level II.
    - HCPCS level I codes are based on AMA Current Procedural Terminology (CPT) because this subsystem mainly represents medical procedures or services by health care professionals.
    - HCPCS level II codes have a broad range. These codes can cover services supplies such as procedures (e.g., screening procedures for TB, head imaging, fall risk assessment, urgent care visits, etc.), services (e.g., ambulance services, hearing services, vision services, etc.), supplies (both medical and surgical), specific health care items such as durable medical equipment (e.g., wheelchairs, etc.), and medications (e.g., chemotherapy drugs, etc.).

Verify insurance and eligibility in the EHR.

The EHR specialist is important to the patient insurance verification and eligibility check for a health care organization. Following verified system access to a specific patient's EHR, the specialist utilizes system features to scan and verify insurance information, reviewing it for accuracy and identifying input errors. Using integrated insurance eligibility and verification tools, the status of patient coverage can be validated to be active with any applicable coinsurance. Verification should be coordinated with billing and insurance companies for validation. Documentation should be recorded to identify validation processes for future data retrieval. Compliance with regulations (HIPAA) and organizational policies is important to maintain through this entire process.

Obtain and document authorizations in the EHR.

Obtaining and documenting prior authorizations in the EHR allows for expedited care delivery. Prior authorization is a strategy used by many insurance companies to ensure that patients receive the most cost-effective care and medications to address their clinical situations. Obtaining and maintaining current authorizations allows for health care providers to easily request authorizations electronically, reducing the time to receipt, approval, and care implementation.

Provide estimated patient costs.

Provision of patient cost information is part of a health care organization's financial transparency and patient engagement initiatives. Estimation of costs for anticipated health care procedures requires taking into account the patient's insurance for covered services addressing deductibles, copayments, coinsurance, and insurance coverage limits. Cost estimation tools can also assist calculation of cost estimation. These tools can be located within the EHR system or retrieved from an outside source. Identification of out-of-pocket costs is an important piece of this estimation, as it can be used by the patient as one of the factors in deciding whether or not to have a procedure. Collaboration with the billing team or insurance company can assist in accuracy of the estimated patient cost.

Navigate the EHR to provide patient statements.

Patient statement information can be retrieved from the features designed to manage the patient account and statements. Following the log-in and authentication, accessing the billing or financial components of the EHR software is necessary. It is necessary to access information for a specific patient by identification, date of birth, or other unique identifiers in the system. A statement can then be generated, which includes recent transactions, outstanding balances, and billing/payment history. Reviewing the statement for accuracy and making changes (edits) may be required for an accurate accounting or up-to-date accounting of activities. These can be generated in paper or electronic format. Adhering to compliance regulations for providing such statements must always be noted such as HIPAA and billing policies, procedures, and regulations.

Collect and post payments to a patient's account.

Accuracy of both collection and posting of payments is important to maintain proper financial records. This task can also be overseen by medical billing staff but may be part of the EHR specialist responsibility in a small health care organization or clinic. Payment integration can provide a seamless way for payments to be input, secured, and tracked by the EHR system. There are software programs that facilitate debit/credit card payment input, contactless payments, bank transfer payments, and so on, as one-time or recurring payments for health care services rendered. It is critical for the EHR specialist to understand how billing is managed and the accounting and billing capabilities (including integration of other systems) of the EHR system in use by an organization in order for claims to be properly processed for reimbursement.

Regulatory Compliance (15% of Exam; 15 Items)

Adhere to professional standards of care as they pertain to health records.

Adhering to professional standards of care require the EHR specialist to adhere to privacy and confidentiality (HIPAA); accurately record and update patient records to maintain data accuracy and integrity; ensure and implement security protocols to safeguard against cyber threats, breaches, and unauthorized access to the various health care record components; maintain ethical use of information to avoid unauthorized sharing or exploitation of the EHR; work to achieve interoperability and seamless transmission of validated and approved patient information; monitor compliance through training and emphasize adherence to protocols and standards for data access, with prompt attention to policy deviation by organizational individuals; and educate patients about their EHR rights and the importance of being an active participant in the management of their health records through accurate updates.

Maintain confidentiality and security of protected health information (PHI) in compliance with the HIPAA Privacy Rule, the Health Information Technology for Economic and Clinical Health (HITECH) Act, and facility policy.

Confidentiality and security of protected health information is critical for the safety of the patient as well as the organization. The following ways ensure these securities:

- Audit trails maintain audit logs, which track who is accessing information, when information is accessed, and for what specific purpose. It is imperative to have a regular review schedule for these audit trails to address unauthorized access quickly.
- Access controls ensure that only persons within the organization with a designated role have access to specific information. Job role information access should be standardized with strong authentication mechanisms.
- Encryption is to be used when sending information that contains PHI to other facilities or remote vendors. This is the process of protecting information on transmission to another designated individual or entity through the use of mathematical models to scramble the information when sent. Only individuals with the key to unscramble the information can access it upon receiving it.
- Breach response plans assign roles and responsibilities for responding to any breach of critical information within an organization. An organizational breach plan should do the following:
    1. Define what constitutes a breach for the organization (e.g., ransomware, phishing, etc.).
    2. Identify who is a member of the breach response team and what their designated roles are to be in relationship to the specific breach.

3. Identify a contact list of essential individuals to be notified, which can include regulatory agencies, legal counsel, cloud service providers, and cybersecurity consultants and experts used by the organization.
4. Formulate alternative effective communication plans in case technological communication is not available. It is imperative that these communications are confidential and only reach the intended person. Have prewritten statements that address various breaches that can be used. Having these available allows time for careful deliberation with legal counsel and others to ensure that the wording does not incite hysteria and produce unwanted confrontations with stakeholders and patients.
5. Initiate the plan for the specific cybersecurity incidents identified. Ensure that each step of the plan is followed specifically and in the proper sequence.

- The HITECH Act is part of the American Recovery and Reinvestment Act (ARRA). Breaches (unauthorized access, acquisition, and/or disclosure of PHI) must follow HITECH Act requirements. Prompt notification is required when there is retrieval of impermissible information per the HIPAA Breach Notification Rule (45 CFR, Part 164, Subpart D). The EHR specialist should also be aware of what does not constitute a breach of PHI, or exceptions, which are (a) unintentional acquisition, access, or PHI use in good faith by an authorized person (e.g., a nurse opens a patient's chart in error when checking orders from a physician; if this was intentional to review the record [opening a record of an important hospitalized person to poke around and see what it contains], this violates the acquisition rule); (b) inadvertent disclosure of PHI information to another authorized person in the organization (e.g., a nurse inadvertently sends radiology findings to the incorrect physician, who informs them of the error and deletes this information); and (c) the unauthorized person receiving the information is unable to retain the PHI information received (e.g., information returned by email as unable to be sent).
- Maintain current policies related to management of the EHR and PHI. There should be a regular schedule for policy review, along with a committee of various individuals to ensure compliance with regulations and procedures.

- Training must be initiated on a designated schedule (usually annually following initial onboard training for new employees), and awareness must be regularly emphasized to maintain a level of attentiveness regarding safeguarding PHI by employees.

Educate others regarding compliance with best practices to safeguard electronic information and assist with enforcement of compliant behaviors.

Education of others not only involves designated training sessions but one-on-one intermittent reviews to promote best practices. The EHR specialist serves to keep all updated-on policies and protocols on a daily basis as individuals interact with the EHR. Enforcement is not just formal reporting but intermittent reminders to keep employees within legal parameters for accessing the patient record. They serve to maintain compliant behaviors, which include not sharing passwords for access to records, locking designated record rooms, and only accessing patient data if there is a need to know. They remind and report when necessary to promote enforcement of disciplinary actions for noncompliant behaviors.

Identify non-compliant behaviors (e.g., sharing passwords, unlocked room) that represent threats to the security of electronic information.

Vigilance in identifying and addressing noncompliant behavior, detection in maintaining secure data and access, are part of the EHR specialist's responsibility. As a member of the collaborative health care team the first component to addressing noncompliant behavior is identification of the behavior by a health care team member. Addressing the specific behavior may include counseling, retraining, and even termination based on organizational policy. This is not an activity that is left to the EHR specialist alone. Usually there is a committee that addresses these breaches by organizational individuals following identification of the noncompliant activity. The EHR specialist is one member of this important committee.

Allocate access controls within the EHR system based on user roles and predetermined privileges.

Access controls are the responsibility of the EHR specialist. These controls ensure that people have access to information needed to perform their job and nothing more. This is determined by role-based access controls (RBAC). The RBAC verify that people have access to tools, applications, and data needed to perform their job effectively and efficiently without interruption. Users can access data to perform actions required based on their role, regulatory requirements, and licensure boundaries. This is important not only for on-boarding but off-boarding employees.

Verify and assist with compliance of access controls (i.e., privileges) within the EHR system.

Access control is critical for organizational online security and EHR safety. The EHR specialist role includes not only verification of who should have access to specific record components but assist with compliance with these controls. In order to achieve this outcome, it is imperative that the EHR specialist is knowledgeable of organizational policies and procedures that form the framework for meeting compliance. This framework clearly identifies who can access specific information as well as disciplinary actions and sanctions for infractions. Access control verification (e.g., user roles, permissions, and restrictions) should be conducted routinely to protect data and comply with organizational and governmental requirements.

De-identify protected health information (PHI).

PHI must be de-identified or anonymized for certain activities such as use in research studies, policy assessments, and specific reports. The information must be de-identified so that individuals cannot be determined from the data nor can they be re-identified from the data. HIPAA compliance must be adhered to for de-identification. Methods that are HIPAA compliant are Expert Determination and Safe Harbor:

- Expert Determination is a method for removing or de-identifying information to make it no longer recognizable as belonging to any individual. It requires a HIPAA-covered entity to obtain an opinion from an individual who has the appropriate knowledge and experience with scientific and statistical principles and methods to de-identify information. The level of expertise is not specifically identified, but this person must be capable of passing an audit of regulators should the information be requested for investigation.

- Safe Harbor is a method for removing or de-identifying information to make it no longer recognizable as belonging to any individual. It specifically states the identifiable data that must be removed. This designated information includes

"(A) Names

(B) All geographic subdivisions smaller than a state, including street address, city, county, precinct, ZIP code, and their equivalent geocodes, except for the initial three digits of the ZIP code if, according to the current publicly available data from the Bureau of the Census:

(1) The geographic unit formed by combining all ZIP codes with the same three initial digits contains more than 20,000 people; and

(2) The initial three digits of a ZIP code for all such geographic units containing 20,000 or fewer people is changed to 000

(C) All elements of dates (except year) for dates that are directly related to an individual, including birth date, admission date, discharge date, death date, and all ages over 89 and all elements of dates (including year) indicative of such age, except that such ages and elements may be aggregated into a single category of age 90 or older

(D) Telephone numbers

(L) Vehicle identifiers and serial numbers, including license plate numbers

(E) Fax numbers

(M) Device identifiers and serial numbers

(F) Email addresses

(N) Web Universal Resource Locators (URLs)

(G) Social security numbers

(O) Internet Protocol (IP) addresses

(H) Medical record numbers

(P) Biometric identifiers, including finger and voice prints

(I) Health plan beneficiary numbers

(Q) Full-face photographs and any comparable images

(J) Account numbers

(R) Any other unique identifying number, characteristic, or code, except as permitted by paragraph (c) of this section [Paragraph (c) is presented below in the section "Re-identification"]; and

(K) Certificate/license numbers".

Reference: U.S. Department of Health and Human Services. (2022, October 25). *Guidance regarding methods for de-identification of protected health information in accordance with the Health Insurance Portability and Accountability Act (HIPAA) privacy rule.* https://www.hhs.gov/hipaa/for-professionals/privacy/special-topics/de-identification/index.html

Release protected health information (PHI) in accordance with the HIPAA Privacy Rule and facility policy.

Releasing PHI must be done in such a way as to protect patient privacy while allowing entities with a 'need to know' access to this information (e.g., insurance companies, consulting health care providers for patient care, etc.). This usually starts with a notice of privacy document given to patients to make them aware of organizational policies and procedures regarding this information. This Notice of Privacy Practice (NPP) is in plain language so that it can be understood by individuals who have various educational levels. Some PHI uses and disclosures may be allowed without patient authorization. These can include information in response to (a) public health authorities for required reporting, (b) law enforcement, and (c) court orders.

Participate in internal audits of the EHR (e.g., consent forms, release of information forms, signature on file).

Participation in internal audits will usually occur at predesignated times (e.g., quarterly, semi-annually, or annually). These audits are done to validate the completeness of information and validate that forms are complete with all required signatures. Consent forms must be validated as containing all required information inclusive of accurate procedure and signatures appropriately dated. Signatures validate that the patient has received informed consent for the procedure inclusive of procedure understanding, risks and benefits, and alternatives. Release of information forms verify that the patient gave consent for information to be released to a specific entity or provider. Random data retrieval on a scheduled basis identifies that the organization and staff are compliant with all required components of the EHR and that they are complete.

Comply with regulations regarding the use of abbreviations in the EHR system.

Abbreviation standardization must be developed by the organization and comply with organizations such as the Joint Commission and the Institute for Safe Medication Practices (ISMP). The intent of these lists is to minimize errors that could result in patient harm.

- The Joint Commission has a list of Do Not Use abbreviations it has developed to promote patient safety. This list applies to all medication-related orders whether they are handwritten or preprinted:
  - U, u (unit) which can be mistaken for zero "o" the number "4" or "cc". Instead: write out the word "unit."
  - IU (international unit) which can be mistaken for intravenous "IV" or the number ten "10". Instead: write out "international unit."
  - Q.D., QD, q.d., qd (daily) can be mistaken for each other. Instead: write out "daily."
  - Q.O.D., QOD, q.o.d, qod (every other day) where the period after the "Q" and the "O" can be mistaken for "I". Instead: write out "every other day."

- Trailing zero (X.0 mg) use can result in the decimal point being missed in medication orders. Instead: write X mg.
- Lack of leading zero (.X mg) can result in missing the decimal point. Instead: write 0.X mg).
- MS can mean morphine sulfate or magnesium sulfate. Instead: write out "morphine sulfate."
- MSO4 and MgSO4 can be confused for one another. Instead: write out "morphine sulfate."

Reference: The Joint Commission. (n.d.). *Do Not Use list fact sheet.* https://www.jointcommission.org/resources/news-and-multimedia/fact-sheets/facts-about-do-not-use-list/

- The ISMP has a list of abbreviations, symbols and dose designations that are identified as being frequently misinterpreted and resulted in medication errors that have caused patient harm. These have been developed through the ISMP National Medication Errors Reporting Program (ISMP MERP). This program allows for health care provider confidential reporting of medication errors and near misses (a situation or event that could have potentially caused harm but did not—a close call that did not result in patient harm as a result of interventional circumstances by the provider or patient). Reporting is not required, and participation in this program is voluntary. The ISMP list contains abbreviations, the intended meaning, misinterpretations that may occur, and corrections. A complete table can be found at https://www.ismp.org/sites/default/files/attachments/2017-11/Error%20Prone%20Abbreviations%202015.pdf.

Initiate down-time procedures related to the EHR (e.g., data recovery).

Downtime is when a computer system, server, or network is not accessible for input or retrieval of information. Downtime can be planned, such as for routine maintenance, or unplanned, caused by a power failure, failure of organization or non organization (offsite) hardware, or hacker attacks. System issues can include updates, rebooting, or even crashes. In all of these scenarios it is necessary to have a system that can recover and not lose critical data. There must also be components put in place to allow data retrieval and minimize disruption to care activities. Downtime is an important part of organizational technology health. The EHR specialist is key to identifying downtime situations and addressing them in order to have the least impact on productivity and revenue. Scheduled maintenance must be done at times that allows the least disruption, which is usually during nighttime hours or when clinics have the least number of patients or are closed for patient services. Preparation and notification are important for scheduled activities that require downtime. Additional onsite or remote personnel may be required and the EHR specialist is responsible for working with the IT department to facilitate a smooth downtime transition to full recovery and system re-initiation. Downtime documentation must be done by the specialist that follows organization policy. This documentation may include how downtime was communicated to all affected personnel, alternate processes put in place for continued care delivery and data capture, how charges were captured for all activities requiring compensation, how systems were returned (brought back up) to full capacity, and how EHR components completed during the downtime period were returned to the system once it was 'live' or back in full working capacity. Recovery will also include validation for retrieval of data into the EHR system following restoration for all entries made during the downtime situation.

Comply with the requirements of EHR incentive programs.

Requirements of EHR incentive programs allow health care providers to be compensated for implementation and upgrading of their software based on meeting certain criteria. In 2022 the Medicaid Promoting Interoperability Program ended. The program is currently known as the Medicare Promoting Interoperability Program for eligible hospitals and critical access hospitals (CAHs). All participants are now required to use the 2015 edition, Certified Electronic Health Record Technology (CEHRT), which was not a prior requirement. In 2022 reporting requirements for the Medicare Promoting Interoperability program mandated use of the CEHRT. An eligible hospital or critical access hospital (CAH) must use the 2015 Edition CEHRT for the full EHR reporting period. The CEHRT improves interoperability through the adoption of new and updated vocabulary and content standards, includes "application access" certification criteria, supports patient electronic access to health information, and includes a revised view, download, and transmit criterion. Hospitals attesting to the Medicare Promoting Interoperability Program for 2023 are scored on four objectives and their measures which include: "(a) electronic prescribing, (b) health information exchange, (c) provider to patient exchange, and (d) public health and clinical data exchange" (Centers for Medicare & Medicaid Services, 2023). They must also attest to "(a) security risk analysis measure, (b) Safety Assurance Factors for EHR Resilience (SAFER) Guides measure, (c) actions to limit or restrict the compatibility or interoperability of CEHRT attestation, and (d) Office of the National Coordinator for Health Information Technology (ONC) Direct Review Attestation" (Centers for Medicare & Medicaid Services, 2023). Having electronic measures in place and a system that is structured to capture all required data for the Medicare Promoting Interoperability Program will facilitate successful incentive recovery.

Reference: Centers for Medicare & Medicaid Services. (2023, September 6). *2022 Medicare Promoting Interoperability Program requirements.* https://www.cms.gov/regulations-guidance/promoting-interoperability/2022-medicare-promoting-interoperability-program-requirements

Reporting (10% of Exam; 10 Items)

Run and execute standardized financial reports (e.g., aging, carriers, financial guarantor, relative value, cost of procedures, prospective payment systems).

The EHRS is critical to effective EHR management in an organization's medical office. It is crucial that medical reports are accurately retrieved (run) in order to report correct data for current and future activities and financial recovery from outside payors. Standardized financial reports are retrieved from databases on a set schedule and/or intermittently as needed to address the status of an organization's financial health. Various reports may include the following:

- Aging reports provide information about outstanding receivables accounts. This allows for identification of monies still owed the organization and the amount of time they have been unpaid (30 days past due, 60 days past due, etc.).

- Carriers reports focus on payments received from insurance companies (insurance carriers). This will give specific monies received from these carriers based on billing.
- Financial guarantor reports identify critical information about obligations of guarantors, which include entities or individuals that provide a guarantee of payment for services. These can be debt repayment or obligation fulfillment by the patient or other party (e.g., insurance, parent, guardian, etc.). These reports include key information about the guarantor's financial position and the terms of the guarantee. This type of report helps investors evaluate guarantee sufficiency.
- The relative value report is a fitness report of an organization. It looks at the organization's assets (worth) compared to the value of similar assets. This report will compare a company's value to industry peers.
- Cost of procedure reports allow an organization to identify its cost compared to others. It also allows patients and clients to view procedure costs in order to make more informed decisions.
  - According to the Centers for Medicare and Medicaid Services, as of January 1, 2021, all U.S. hospitals were required to provide a clear and accessible online pricing list to allow persons seeking care to be better informed about items and service costs.
  - Medicare price look-up allows Medicare beneficiaries an opportunity to review national average prices for procedures performed at ambulatory surgical centers and hospital outpatient departments.
  - FAIR health is a nonprofit organization that collects information regarding health care costs and coverage. It has the largest U.S. database of privately billed health insurance claims, which allows for transparency of care costs and insurance information. This site reports benchmarks, trackers (e.g., disease, birth costs, opioid, telehealth), and market reports. The FAIR Health website can be accessed at https://www.fairhealth.com.
- The prospective payment system report is a method used by Medicare to determine the rate of payment for various health care services. In other words, the payment received by the provider is based on a fixed, predetermined amount. Its intent is to regulate payments to providers to ensure fair and

efficient compensation for services rendered. The payment received by the provider is determined by the classification system of that specific service.

- The Inpatient Prospective Payment System is a reimbursement framework used for care delivered by acute care hospitals. Using the Diagnosis Related Group (DRG) categorization, Medicare Part A (covers a hospital stay, skilled nursing facility, hospice care delivery, and some home health care) fee-for-service payment bundles care components and costs for that care.
    - Diagnosis Related Group (DRG) is a specific document that gives weights to specific diagnoses. This identifies the average resources used to treat a specific illness or diagnosis for Medicare patients. Each DRG has a base payment weight that reflects average resources used to treat that specific diagnosis for Medicare patients. If the patient diagnosis is more complex, this would require more resources, which would result in a higher payment rate and more monetary return to the organization for care.
    - A Disproportionate Share Hospital (DSH) Adjustment provides for hospitals serving a higher proportion of low-income patients and those individuals without insurance. These hospitals receive additional monies through an increase in Medicare payment.
- The Post-Acute Care (PAC) Prospective Payment System (PPS) reports retrieve information related to proposed payment for Medicare-covered post-acute care hospital services. These services provide care following acute post hospital inpatient services that could be supplied by an inpatient rehabilitation facility (IRF), long-term care hospital (LTCH), skilled nursing facility (SNF), or home health agency (HHA). Each facility has its own Medicare fee-for-service plan that identifies payment for designated services.

- Clinical reports can be run for specific patient outcomes. These allow for identification of care delivery and outliers that may be outside the cost identified by specific entities for care delivery. These reports can be run for any number of specific identifiers, which include but are not limited to patient diagnosis, procedures performed (inpatient or outpatient specific), or health care provider administering patient care.

Run and execute standardized clinical reports to track patient outcomes (e.g., by diagnosis, by procedure, by provider) for the support of continuity of care.

The EHR is an individualized record of a patient's specific care delivery. In order to identify trends and track patient outcomes, data must be retrieved from several records and viewed in an analytical summary component. Aggregation of data allows for review of patterns in diagnoses treated at specific times of year, procedures performed at a facility, and provider-specific information who work at a facility (number of patients seen, type of patients seen, etc.) over a specific period of time. Reviewing data allows for the organization to provide care to all individuals that is complete, consistent, and connected based on data retrieval, analysis, and review over designated periods of time.

Generate ad hoc financial reports using fields in the EHR system.

An ad hoc financial report is one that is obtained on demand. It is obtained from financial records in order to fulfill a need for specific information in a designated report. Retrieval of this information is outside the usually scheduled data retrieval schedule based on necessity and need. It will require identification of specific fields or cells for retrieval in order to perform analyses as requested. A field is the fundamental building block of a data system and serves to identify information location. The requester must be specific and detailed in what is needed for the report in order to retrieve data that addresses the specific need.

Generate ad hoc clinical reports using fields in the EHR system.

An ad hoc clinical report is one that is obtained on demand. It is obtained from patient health records in order to fulfill a need for specific information in a designated report. Retrieval of this information is outside the usually scheduled data retrieval schedule based on necessity and need. It will require identification of specific fields or cells for retrieval in order to perform analyses as requested. A field is the fundamental building block of a data system and serves to identify information location. The requester must be specific and detailed in what is needed for the report in order to retrieve data that addresses the specific need.

Generate statistical reports for quality improvement (QI) measures, productivity, metrics, and research.

Statistical reports serve to enhance the services of an organization through analyses of collected data. Data is retrieved based on identified specific information and systematically analyzed to describe and evaluate characteristics of the specific topic under investigation. The form of analysis will depend on the purpose of the retrieved data. Quality improvement serves to standardize processes for care delivery, which reduces variation in care delivery to achieve and improve patient outcomes and organizational outcomes as well. Statistical reports promote improved productivity, which in turn can improve financial security for the organization. This data can be compared or statistically analyzed to determine research outcomes to identify if a difference exists between specific components (e.g., the difference between patient care outcomes based on medicines prescribed for high cholesterol) or if there is a relationship between specific components (e.g., the relationship between patient age and breast-feeding outcome for clinic patients).

Compile data from the EHR for external reporting (e.g., for Meaningful Use / Quality Payment Program [QPP]).

This is retrieval of data for compilation and analyses to determine organizational ability to meet specific external regulations.

Medicare Promoting Interoperability Program Requirements (prior Meaningful Use)

- Interoperability promotion is the minimum standard for the EHR. It identifies how patient data exchange can occur between providers, insurers, and patients. Reports must verify that the organization is complying with these requirements. CMS 2023 requirements are identified:

"Eligible hospitals and critical access hospitals (CAHs) attesting to CMS will be required to report on four scored objectives.

6. Electronic Prescribing
7. Health Information Exchange
8. Provider to Patient Exchange
9. Public Health and Clinical Data Exchange

Medicare Promoting Interoperability Program participants must also attest to the following:

- Security Risk Analysis measure
- Safety Assurance Factors for EHR Resilience (SAFER) Guides measure
- Actions to limit or restrict the compatibility or interoperability of CEHRT attestation
- Office of the National Coordinator for Health Information Technology (ONC) Direct Review Attestation" (Centers for Medicare and Medicaid Services, 2023).

Reference: Centers for Medicare & Medicaid Services. (2023, September 6). *2022 Medicare Promoting Interoperability Program Requirements*. https://www.cms.gov/regulations-guidance/promoting-interoperability/2022-medicare-promoting-interoperability-program-requirements

QPP

Quality Payment Program (QPP) goals are to improve care quality and safety for all individuals and reduce clinician administrative burden. These goals serve to promote more focused person-centered care by health care personnel, thereby improving health outcomes. QPP has two payment tracks: the Merit-based Incentive Program (MIP) and Advanced Alternative Payment Model (APM) (see Figure 11.1).

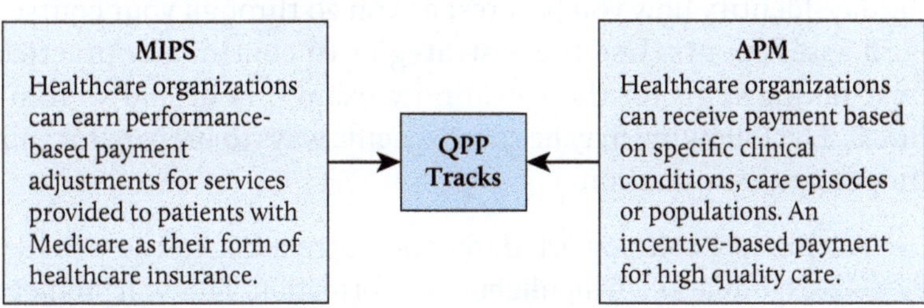

FIGURE 11.1 QPP tracks.

Verify the accuracy of generated reports prior to distribution (e.g., check for errors).

It is important the EHR specialist can design reports for their specifically designated purpose. This is the first step in verifying report accuracy. One must know the type of report to generate before knowing what data is needed for retrieval and statistical analyses. For example, coded data can eliminate ambiguity as it is numerical in nature and validated through an internal audit for accuracy when generating a production report. Another example is a production by procedure report in which a CPT code from the EHR can be used in report generation. This data-driven report retrieves data from the EHR to provide insight into performance and efficiency of specific health care procedures or functions. This allows for metrics optimization and error reduction. Data input accuracy is key to report accuracy. The integrity of the health care record will produce accurate data verification prior to retrieval, which is the best way to verify that the report obtained is correct.

Preparation for the CEHRS Examination

Just thinking of preparing for a certification examination can increase your heart rate. It can be a daunting task. The key to success is to be adequately prepared and confident in your ability to be successful.

Preparation starts from day 1 of the first course you take, up to the day you sit for the examination. Preparation is continuous and includes all course work taken for completion of your program. Study, review information often, and prepare yourself day by day. Identify how you best test as you go through your courses and assessments. Use these strategies to continually practice test-taking skills for the 110-minute exam (1 hour and 50 minutes). The following may be some specific ways to prepare for this important examination:

- Review coursework daily and correlate it to the CEHRS examination to highlight key information. This will promote information retention and improve problem-solving skills.

- Review the content examination outline, which can be found online. Highlight areas that you feel need the most focus of your study as you review the list.
- Retrieve and organize your study material. Identify whether you will focus on electronic materials or hard-copy materials based on how you prefer to learn and study. These resources can assist you in snatching bits of time and expediting study (carrying an electronic study aid can be used as you wait for the kids to get out of school, you are stuck in traffic, etc.). This step will also facilitate reinforcement of knowledge gained.
- Develop a study plan to promote successful time management. Components to include should address content review, practice examinations, and identification of areas needing specific attention for success. Goals should be realistic and attainable. Develop a schedule and stick to it as this will be the best way to ensure you have enough time to prepare for the examination.
- Use a study group if this facilitates your learning and retention of information and core concepts. Teaching others through repetition and information review and dialogue can help retention and promote you gaining a different perspective on examination content. Using a study group can also keep you motivated and on your study plan task and timeline.
- Take practice tests, preferably in an online format to assist you with electronic testing. This will help you develop ease and comfort with this testing format. Using hard-copy information can certainly assist in identification of areas needing more focused study as well. These can promote improvement of test-taking strategies (identification of key words in a question and how to select the most correct response). Be sure to review the rationale for correct as well as incorrect answers.
- Practice time management while testing by simulating an actual examination format. Set yourself up as you would be in a real testing environment (be alone, remove distractions, set a timer, take it while in a real test mentality). This will help you identify if you need to improve time to completion by reducing test item time to answer. Thinking into the question can promote incorrect selection by rationalizing

each option as potentially correct. Work to identify the time you need to select an option based on key words or phrases in a question (e.g., What are they really looking for? What is the most correct answer?)

- Use positive affirmations. These are positive phrases or statements that can be written, stated aloud, or repeated in thought to oneself to maintain confidence and optimism. Positive affirmations can decrease stress and improve overall well-being, which can lead to improved academic performance and a better outlook for examination success.
- Practice breathing exercises for relaxation. Taking a few slow, deep breaths while in a comfortable position can reduce stress and promote well-being. There are various breathing exercises for anxiety and stress relief. Find one you like and practice it regularly.

The examination is administered by the National Healthcareer Association (NHA) at approved test sites across the United States. Examination success is based on meeting the scaled passing score of 390. The scaled score range is 200 to 500. The CEHRS detailed examination outline is identified to assist you in preparation - https://www.nhanow.com/docs/default-source/test-plans/nha_cehrs-test-plan.pdf?sfvrsn=ad996ae5_2.

Various Domains and Sub-Domains That Are Covered by the CEHRS Exam

Domain 1: Non-Clinical Operations (28 Items)

- Verify patient identifiers before documenting in the EHR to ensure information is recorded in the correct chart.
- Collect, record, and continuously update patient information (e.g., demographic information, clinical data, coverages/financial/insurance, guarantors, patient preferences).
- Generate encounter documentation (e.g., admission/face sheet, labels, armbands).
- Retrieve patient information from internal databases (e.g., provider database, financial database) to integrate into a patient's EHR.
- Acquire patient data from external sources (e.g., diagnostic laboratories, ancillary facilities, other healthcare providers, other EHR systems)

- Import information into the EHR from integrated devices (e.g., scanners, fax machines, e-signature pads, cameras).
- Maintain inventory of EHR-related hardware (e.g., e-signature pads, cameras, tablets, mobile devices).
- Coordinate patient flow within the facility (e.g., scheduling, patient registration and verification, check-in/check-out, patient referrals).
- Provide initial and ongoing end-user training of EHR software to maintain competency (e.g., for new hires, upgrades and deployments).
- Share information about updates to EHR software and the implications for workflow.
- Identify data discrepancies within and among multiple EHRs, practice management systems, and other software systems.
- Report or reconcile data discrepancies within and among multiple EHRs, practice management systems, and other software systems.
- Provide support to patients regarding their use of patient portals (e.g., basic introduction, explain utility, grant access, navigation help).

Domain 2: Clinical Operations (32 Items)

- Develop clinical templates for data capture (e.g., by diagnosis, by procedure, by practice).
- Securely transmit and exchange patient data internally and externally (e.g., to pharmacies, other healthcare providers, other agencies) for research, analytics, and continuity of care.
- Review and monitor clinical documentation to ensure completeness and accuracy (e.g., self-review, peer-to-peer).
- Provide point-of-care EHR support (e.g., at-the-elbow, remote) for clinical documentation.
- Input real-time clinical data into the EHR.
- Document patient historic clinical data in the EHR (e.g., medications, immunizations, surgeries).
- Provide support for computerized provider order entry (CPOE).
- Locate and provide patient education materials available within the EHR.
- Navigate the EHR system to retrieve requested patient data.

Domain 3: Revenue Cycle/Finance (15 Items)

- Find codes in databases (e.g., International Statistical Classification of Diseases and Related Health Problems [ICD], Current Procedural Terminology [CPT], and Healthcare Common Procedure Coding System [HCPCS]).
- Navigate the EHR to create a superbill, encounter forms, fee slips, or charge forms.
- Enter the diagnosis and procedure codes billing information (e.g., from a superbill) into the EHR system for claims processing.
- Verify that all diagnoses and procedural descriptions for reimbursement are accurately documented in the EHR.
- Verify insurance and eligibility in the EHR.
- Obtain and document authorizations in the EHR.
- Provide estimated patient costs.
- Navigate the EHR to provide patient statements.
- Collect and post payments to a patient's account.

Domain 4: Regulatory Compliance (15 Items)

- Adhere to professional standards of care as they pertain to health records.
- Maintain confidentiality and security of protected health information (PHI) in compliance with the HIPAA Privacy Rule, the Health Information Technology for Economic and Clinical Health (HITECH) Act, and facility policy.
- Educate others regarding compliance with best practices to safeguard electronic information and assist with enforcement of compliant behaviors.
- Identify non-compliant behaviors (e.g., sharing passwords, unlocked room) that represent threats to the security of electronic information.
- Allocate access controls within the EHR system based on user roles and predetermined privileges (least privilege access).
- Verify and assist with compliance of access controls (i.e., privileges) within the EHR system.
- De-identify protected health information (PHI).
- Release protected health information (PHI) in accordance with the HIPAA Privacy Rule and facility policy.
- Participate in internal audits of the EHR (e.g., consent forms, release of information forms, signature on file).

- Comply with regulations regarding the use of abbreviations in the EHR system.
- Initiate down-time procedures related to the EHR (e.g., data recovery).
- Comply with the requirements of EHR incentive programs.

Domain 5: Reporting (10 Items)

- Run and execute standardized financial reports (e.g., aging, carriers, financial guarantor, relative value, cost of procedures, prospective payment systems).
- Run and execute standardized clinical reports to track patient outcomes (e.g., by diagnosis, by procedure, by provider) for the support of continuity of care.
- Generate ad hoc financial reports using fields in the EHR system.
- Generate ad hoc clinical reports using fields in the EHR system.
- Generate statistical reports for quality improvement (QI) measures, productivity, metrics, and research.
- Compile data from the EHR for external reporting (e.g., for Meaningful Use/Quality Payment Program [QPP]).
- Verify the accuracy of generated reports prior to distribution (e.g., check for errors).

Core/Foundational Knowledge

The following knowledge statements do not represent standalone domains on the CEHRS exam. Rather, these are fundamental skills and necessary knowledge for those who perform specialized tasks within in the electronic health record, which could be used in the context of an assessment item and are being provided for preparation and review purposes.

- Healthcare regulatory agencies (e.g., Centers for Medicare and Medicaid Services [CMS], The Joint Commission [TJC], United States Department of Health and Human Services [HHS]) and their relevance to EHR practices
- Professional standards related to EHR practices (e.g., Centers for Medicare and Medicaid Services [CMS], Health Insurance Portability and Accountability Act [HIPAA], Health

Information Technology for Economic and Clinical Health [HITECH] Act, Meaningful Use/Quality Payment Program [QPP], Systematized Nomenclature of Medicine – Clinical Terms [SNOMED CT])

- Medical terminology
- Basic healthcare finance terminology
- Healthcare systems, settings, and personnel (e.g., facility types, roles, credentials)
- Parts of the EHR (e.g., demographic information, clinical records, medication administration record, diagnoses, laboratory reports, orders, billing information)
- Protected health information (PHI)
- Types and implications for use of health records (e.g., paper or electronic [including app-based/mobile, computer-based, web-based/online])
- Types of healthcare documentation (e.g., Subjective, Objective, Assessment, Plan [SOAP] progress notes, laboratory reports, imaging, operative reports, orders)
- General function(s) and purpose of the EHR (e.g., continuity of care, streamlined care)
- Patient rights and responsibilities
- Interoperability concepts
- Population health concepts

Index

F

About the Author

Dr. Maria Revell started her career as a nurse and moved to incorporate education as her passion for promoting successful careers in the lives of others grew. She has educated nurses in academic and clinical settings from entry level to advanced practice, but ... her quest to enhance student education to improve an individual's self-life as well as the lives of those they touch professionally and personally did not stop there. Education is foundational to the promotion of better lifestyle choices, greater advocacy, and improvement of self-worth. This moved her to expand educational endeavors beyond U.S. borders to include China, Cuba, South Africa, and the Czech Republic. Successful outcomes are important for all seeking to improve their life through education. She has worked with individuals in various interdisciplinary healthcare professions. Her experience in electronic health records includes utilization and review from clinical, educational, and legal perspectives. The desire to specifically improve the lives of those moving into the role of electronic health records specialist through education was the impetus to write this book.

Dr. Revell received her bachelor's degree in nursing from Tuskegee Institute, AL, her master's degree from the University of Alabama, Huntsville, and her doctorate from the University of Alabama, Birmingham. She has published numerous peer-reviewed articles on various topics from technology to patient care. In addition to publications, her passion for education drove her to write grants to support student success. Many have touched her life, as students, colleagues, mentors, friends, and family. They are all an integral part of this current work.

www.ingramcontent.com/pod-product-compliance
Ingram Content Group UK Ltd.
Pitfield, Milton Keynes, MK11 3LW, UK
UKHW021830270726
14058UKWH00001B/72

9 798823 350372